LONGEVITY UNLOCKED

FIT FOR LIFE

The Secret Of Staying Young While Growing Old

NOSHIR N. SANJANA

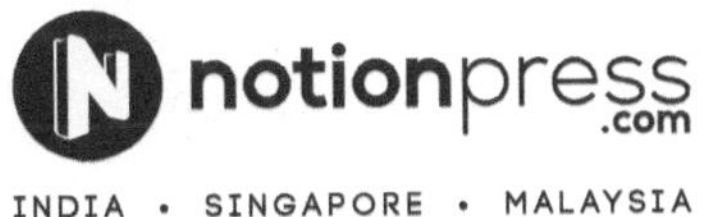

ISBN
Paperback 979-8-89632-475-1
Hardcase 979-8-89929-740-3

AUTHORS NOTE

My purpose in life is to be healthy, happy, and fit. It should be your purpose in life, too.

If you have a deep desire and a strong determination to heal yourself, maximise your health, and live a long, fruitful, and active life:

THIS IS JUST THE BOOK FOR YOU.

Noshir N. Sanjana

Author's qualifications:

Masters in L.B.D.N.

"Looking Busy Doing Nothing."

Bachelor in M.A.B.F.M.

"Metric (SSCE) Appeared, But Failed Miserably."

M.B.B.S.

"Member of Betha Bekaar Society" (Member of the time-wasting association)

After all, your degrees are just a piece of paper. Your education is seen through your behaviour and what you do with your life.

People say nothing is impossible, but I do nothing every day.

There are four things you must do so that you never grow old.

1. Smoke two or three packets of cigarettes every day.

2. Drink one bottle of country liquor every day.

3. Never eat home-cooked food. Eat only pizza, hamburgers, pasta, and instant Maggi noodles every day with dollops of butter and cheese.

4. No need for point number four. Follow the above three points, and you will never grow old. You will meet your maker well before old age! *Aap ka ticket jawani mein hi cut jaayega!*

WELCOME AND INTRODUCTION

This book is a dedication to the journey of life, marked by resilience, good health, and the quest for wellness. It is motivated by personal experiences, enhanced with insight and the wisdom of age, and guided by the desire to share knowledge that can revolutionise lives.

The most important thing for every individual is to love life, and LIVE IT!! It is also important to share knowledge and inspirations by living cordially and in oneness with all.

This book contains chapters on the principles of how to live your life in accordance with natural laws of life, love, friendship, endearment, and modern and ancient science related to good health.

Read the chapter, "Saaro Manas, a good man - The Master Key" and you WILL become the master of your life with more joy, abundance, and love—every single day of your life.

DEDICATION

Dedicated to my very dearest wife Maloo, and my two darling daughters, Zeena and Jennifer, whose strength and love have been steadfast and resolute pillars of vigour and solidity for me.

Their endurance and commitment have made this venture not just possible but also exceedingly fulfilling.

Family isn't about blood. It is about who is willing to hold your hand when you need it most.

ACKNOWLEDGEMENTS

I extend my gratitude to my elder brother Rusi, who lives in New York and is like a father to me. My inspiration in healthy and holistic living, he and his wife, Gover, are exemplars of living well. Their approach to health and fitness, at ages 93 and 92, showcases the potential of a life well-lived, combining the knowledge and philosophy of alternative medicines with the discipline of routine, consistent physical training.

DISCLAIMER

The mission of this book is not just to inform but to enlighten the reader. None of the information is intended as medical advice. This is all from my own studies and research over the years. I stand true to every statement I have written in this book.

I have tried to be accurate and authentic. I have checked and double-checked from what I believe to be true and factual sources. What is in the book is from my own assessment and conclusion, drawing from personal research and experiences rather than professional medical advice.

It is recommended to take professional advice from a medical practitioner or consult your healthcare provider before starting any new treatment or making any changes to treatment.

My goal is to arouse action, motivate, and stimulate the minds of my readers in transforming their lives, and bringing about a healthier world.

Noshir N. Sanjana

CONTENTS

FOREWORD

A journey into the heart of life's golden years, this book addresses the fabric of ageing and wisdom with realistic advice. It advocates a holistic approach to living, merging ancient wisdom with modern breakthroughs, adding life to years rather than years to life.

The Essence of Ageing Gracefully explores the notion of ageing not as a decline but as a new chapter of opportunities and possibilities. Through personal anecdotes and scientific revelations, it highlights the importance of a well-balanced way of living, the role of nutrition, and the power of positive thinking.

Health and Well-being scrutinises the strategies for preserving physical and mental health. It covers a range of topics from heart health to mental alertness, emphasising natural cures, precautionary care, and the significance of happiness, laughter, and love.

Nutrition and Lifestyle focuses on dietary habits and lifestyle choices. It discusses the benefits of traditional diets, the role of superfoods, and the importance of physical activity, offering practical tips for incorporating these into everyday life.

Legacy and Life Lessons reflects on the lessons learned over a lifetime, sharing wisdom on living with purpose, making meaningful connections, and the art of absolution and letting go. It underlines the legacy of resilience, the significance and value of family, and the exhilaration of lifelong enlightenment and learning.

Conclusion and Looking Ahead summarises the key topics and motives of the book and encourages readers to embrace ageing with grace, a curious mind, and optimism.

It calls for a celebration of life at every age, advocating for a future where every individual can live to their fullest capability and greatest expertise.

Age is merely a number.

Do you know the secret to living for 100 years?

Come closer and I'll let you in on the secret.

(Whisper) First, live to 99 years. And then be very, very careful and very, very cautious for the next one year.

But how do I live to 99 years, you ask?

Well, there you are on your own. But I can help you with my suggestions, tips, and recommendations. You can get there and beyond: robust, in fine fettle, and in great shape.

This is no gimmick or unsubstantiated flimsy banter. The intent of this book is simple and straightforward. I want my readers, family, and friends to *add life to their years and not just years to their lives.* Unlike,

Happy P. Sodabottleopenerwala.

Happy was a middle-aged Parsi gentleman. He had heard of Dr Belly Goofy, a famous doctor who held the secret elixir for a very, very long life. Happy decided to get the elixir for himself.

Happy: Doc, I've come for your secret potion, the elixir which will prolong my life to a hundred years.

Dr Belly: Okay, but I need to ask you a few questions. Do you smoke?

Happy: I have never touched a cigarette in my life.

Dr Belly: What about hard liquor? Vodka? Whisky? Beer?

Happy: I have never, ever had a drink. Alcohol will not touch my lips. I don't go to bars either.

Dr Belly: Women? Do you have a lot of women in your life? Are you a skirt chaser?

Happy: (looking shocked) No, never. Don't need any women in my life.

Dr Belly: (advances threateningly towards Happy) You don't smoke. You don't drink. You don't womanise. Your life is not worth living. Then why the bloody hell do you want to live to 100 years? Get out!! No elixir for you.

Thank you.

Noshir

—— CHAPTER ——
1

TWO MASSIVE HEART ATTACKS, BACK TO BACK

I am certain that any person who questions a doctor's financial motive in performing an essential surgery has to make sure he is fully revived from anaesthesia before discussing the expenses involved, etc. when the same doctor has just operated on him.

Sometimes I like to live dangerously. Sometimes danger skirts my life.

One day, in the first week of March 1993, *Brown Girl in the Ring, Tra la la la la,* ♫ ♪ ♫ 𝄞 ♫ ♪ ♫ *There's a brown girl in the ring, Tra la la la la la* filled the car as Maloo, my wife, my own *sugar in a plum*, was singing to Boney M's 70s song. We were driving from the airport to our house in Kalina, the car speakers were on full blast, and I was tapping the beat on the steering wheel. Life was glorious.

All of a sudden, I felt a sharp jolt of pain in my chest, and I gasped. The pain travelled to my left shoulder and engulfed my whole left arm. I felt a steamy perspiration on my forehead, and my fingers gripped the wheel instead of the light tapping. Maloo turned to me, my *sugar in a plum* immediately sensed something was very wrong.

We were near the Vakola pipeline. At the military junction, Maloo told me to turn left towards the Air India medical clinic at the old airport, instead of taking a right to Kalina. I hesitated for a few seconds, but due to the pain, I turned left. By the time we reached the Air India old airport gate, the pain subsided. I turned the wheel as if to make a U-turn instead of going through the gate when Maloo guessed what I was doing. "We are already here. Might as well see a doctor," she said.

In the clinic, I walked directly to Dr Puri's office. There were other patients waiting to see him, but seeing the look on my face, he guided me straight to the couch. Dr Puri gave me an injection and placed a couple of Sorbitrates and aspirins under my tongue. Before I knew what was happening, I was on my way to Hinduja Hospital in Mahim in the Air India ambulance with Maloo and an intern in tow.

Our old neighbour and friend, Srinivasan Sitapatti, was at the reception in Hinduja Hospital. In minutes he got me admitted to the ICU. Cardiologist Dr Jamshed Dalal attended to me. Meanwhile, Srinivasan called my daughters. Soon they were by my side, consulting and talking to all the attending doctors. The doctors decided to do an angiography on me the next day.

I thought all my pain would be gone, but I had the same excruciating pain in the chest and left arm during the angiography procedure the next day. I was sure it was another heart attack. And it was—a second heart attack. During the angiography, Dr Jamshed Dalal found three major blockages in my main arteries: two 90% blockages and one 100%.

The top surgeon, Dr Nitin Mandke, was called in for a consultation by my daughters and Dr Jamshed Dalal.

The prognosis was that I required a triple bypass surgery. When I heard that, I wanted to give everyone the slip and run home. I was in good health and only 52 years young. I decided I did not need any surgery, definitely not a bypass. It was common knowledge among the uninformed like me that open-heart surgery was a moneymaking racket.

But Maloo, my two daughters, Dr Jamshed Dalal, and Dr Nitin Mandke convinced me that the surgery was absolutely essential and very, very crucial for my continued well-being. What could I do? I convinced myself that Dr Jamshed Dalal was a Zoroastrian Parsi and would not mislead me. So, the surgery date was fixed for two days later.

The hospital needed a few bottles of blood for my open-heart surgery. A notice was put up at our scheduling office and the airport operations office that Noshir Sanjana was to go under the knife in Hinduja Hospital and would require some voluntary blood donors, irrespective of the blood type. Irrespective of blood type? Were they going to pump in a cocktail of blood types into my veins? No, they were planning to stock their blood bank.

Soon there was a long line of my crew members, some crew scheduling officers, our office peon, and even one of our office stenographers, waiting and wanting to donate blood for me. I needed four to five bottles of blood during my procedure, but the Hinduja Hospital pathology lab and blood bank were more than happy to collect dozens and dozens of bottles of blood from my friends under my name. Finally, my best friend Ramesh Angle realised the situation and stood at the pathology lab and turned away all the would-be donors, with many thanks on behalf of me and my family.

By the time the surgery date rolled around, my sister Lily flew down in a mad rush from Toronto. My uncles, my aunts, my cousins, my nephews, all my neighbours from Golden View, and some ex-neighbours from the Air India colony were all there in support of my wife and my daughters.

A double team of doctors, nurses, anesthesiologists, and surgeons stood by for any adverse, untoward emergencies since I had a second heart attack during the angiogram. The triple bypass surgery took more than half a day. The next thing I remember is lying half-awake, very dazed, and disoriented in the recovery room. I felt like a science experiment—enveloped in a bubble, full of tubes, a couple of holes in my chest for the pipes, needles, an oxygen mask, electronic connections, machines, bandages, and other paraphernalia all around and into me. I remember asking my surgeon, Dr Mandke, in the recovery room how many more years I could expect my heart to beat after the bypass surgery. He told me the operation was a total success and confidently gave me another 10 years.

Ten more years? Wow! Seemed like a long, long time ahead of me. I calculated—eight more years of flying, plus a couple of years of retired life sounded great. The only thing that worried me was that I did not have a nest egg accumulated for my family after me.

After the recovery room, I was wheeled to the ICU. Dr Mandke came over one more time to see me before leaving for the day. He was trailed by a couple of junior doctors and two nurses.

I blame the drugs and the anaesthesia, but I blurted out a question that had been niggling at me since before the surgery, "Doctor, please tell me, did I need the surgery, or did you need the money?"

Dr. Mandke was stunned, but he realised I was heavily sedated. He came back with his return volley. "Have you seen my new villa? Somebody has to pay for it, young man! Your heart is in the right place. Thank you for your generosity." The junior doctors and nurses had a good laugh, but I could not even chuckle—it hurt to laugh. Dr Mandke noted my wince with a smug grin. With great dignity, he left the ICU. I thought I had lost my cardiologist and the very best heart surgeon in India, forever. He had just saved my life, and I had questioned his motives. But an hour later, his doctor anesthesiologist wife, who had been there for the entire heart surgery procedure, apologised to me for her husband's remark about the villa. "We have no villa. We live in an apartment," she explained. She was charming, very compassionate, and understanding. Now I blamed her, thinking maybe she had messed up and given me an extra dose of anesthesia, which is why I spoke to her husband the way I did. But I just mumbled, "It's okay. I don't have a villa either." And hoped the ceasefire truce had been made.

I was in a lot of pain. My chest seemed scorched and felt as if there was a huge rock on top of it. My entire left leg hurt, and it felt like a hive of bees was continually stinging me. I did not know that my surgeon had lacerated, removed, and again stitched up three feet of my vein from my left leg and two feet of veins or arteries from either side of my chest. The stitches were not nylon thread or any fabric threads. They were made with finely thinned real cat guts that got infected two weeks after I was discharged. Thick yellowish pus mixed with blood oozed in and on my chest. I was back in the hospital where the stitches were removed and restitched. With different cat guts, I hoped. My sternum bone and my ribs were clipped together with six metal clips. I did not know it then, but the clips would set alarms ringing at airport security checks, and I had to show them a certificate from the doctor and Hinduja Hospital that carried a waiver. Dr Mrs Mandke increased the painkillers in my system and sedated me enough to relax my body and mind.

I dozed off for many hours. Between waking up and dozing off, it was very comforting to see my sister Lily, my Maloo, Zeena, Jennifer, and Mehernosh in turns, one at a time. A personal, special ICU nurse stayed round the clock by my side.

The next day it seemed as if I had bounced back a bit, but the pain continued to be excruciating. There was a continuous stream of Air India friends visiting me. I spun a story to some of them to give me some hundred-rupee notes to tip the ward boys. Very soon, I had a stack of hundred-rupee notes. In the afternoon, I managed to bribe a ward boy who was mopping the floor. I addressed him as *Dikra Ramu* and asked him to purchase a couple of strips of Brufen 600s for me with the hundred-rupee notes I had stashed. I did not know that ward boys dispensed medical advice, too. He sidled closer to me and mumbled that Brufen 600 would not cut it. What I needed was some ganja, and he would be happy to procure some for me. I was tempted, oh so tempted! But I disappointed Ramu by sticking with Brufen 600. Two hours later, I swallowed a handful of painkillers, Brufen 600s. I was on cloud nine, and the rock from my chest had lifted.

I must have been on a high. The same evening, I slipped out of the ICU pushing a steel stand on wheels holding the saline bottle, to meet all my family members in the guest waiting room. This caused a bit of an alarm, hysteria, and frenzy inside and outside the ICU, but I was thrilled to see all my family at the same time. However, I came down to earth when, two days later, I had internal bleeding due to the Brufen 600.

Later, I heard that they had put up a big notice on different Air India office noticeboards that no one was allowed to visit me in the hospital as I was very hyper and overactive. That put a damper on my social life in the hospital.

A week later, around mid-afternoon, on 12th March 1993, I was discharged from the hospital.

A truly history-making date for discharge: at around the same time I was being driven in the ambulance from Hinduja Hospital in Mahim to Kalina, a series of bomb blasts were rocking Bombay, in various locations. Hotels, office buildings, banks, petrol pumps, and markets were bombed and blasted. A series of 12 terrorist bombing attacks took place on that day in Bombay. Two hundred and 57 people were killed, and another 14 hundred were injured and hospitalised. A total of 13 RDX car bombs with shrapnel had been used. It was the darkest and saddest day for Bombayites.

The Almighty blessed my family and me. I survived a heart attack while driving. I survived 90 per cent blockages and a triple bypass. And I survived a few strips of Brufen 600 from Dikra Ramu. Lastly, I survived 13 different RDX bomb blasts while I was in an ambulance on the road in North Bombay. I later learned that the closest we came to danger was when we drove past Fishermen's Colony where grenades were thrown.

I was on extended sick leave from Air India and away from flying duties. My unbearable, agonizingly intensive pains and sleepless nights led to a depressive frame of mind. I was down in the dumps, tossed and turned, imagining that I would have become a vegetable and thus a nuisance to my near and dear ones. But worry does not take away tomorrow's problems; it takes away today's peace of mind, losing belief that this was only a bend and not an end.

I acknowledged that I did not have the best genes. My father had suffered his first heart attack at the same age. To our utter sorrow, he passed away at the age of 64 after surviving another three or four major death-defying heart attacks.

My mother passed away at the tender age of 55 after a long battle with pleurisy and lung cancer. She suffered for over a year in excruciating pain due to water formation in her lungs leading to cancer. The whole family was in deep anguish as we grieved her death. Our only solace was that she was not in pain anymore. We drew comfort in the thought that my mother now walked with the Almighty.

I began to ponder my short longevity of ten years. I had eight years to retire and nothing to show in my bank account. I had to provide for my family as urgently as possible. I still had to get my two beautiful daughters married. I also needed to save and make a little nest egg for me and my wife post-retirement, if I lived to see retirement, or for my wife after I was gone. I had to find ways to take extra good care of my new heart. I had to start saving as much as I could and raise my bank balance. All these days I had a *Saving? What's that!?* attitude to life. That had to change. I needed to live more than the expected 10 years. Besides following my cardiologist's advice and taking the prescribed medication, I would have to forge my own path to stay healthy. I started reading books on how to be heart-healthy. What to eat, what to avoid. I read about herbal and Ayurveda products. On my travels, I visited pharmacies in London and New York that advertised and sold herbal products.

The information we gathered in those days, the days before we even knew the word internet, was a drop in the ocean. Yet we devoured the whole new world it opened, and the many doors it opened up for better health and longevity.

My uncle Naval Sanjana, my brother Rusi, and I started reading and researching everything to comprehend ways and means to gain better health. Soon, we became well-versed and quite knowledgeable in the world of Ayurveda, alternative medications, and the world of herbal magic.

My maternal aunt, Perin Naval Sanjana, who lived in Toronto, Canada, was declared by her cardiologist to have a very weak heart. She was in her sixties. Her husband, my uncle, Naval Sanjana, did not give up hope. Without consulting the doctor, he put my aunt on mega doses of Coenzyme Q10 daily (CoQ10) 400 mg daily. This was followed by the maximum strength of Omega 3 fish oils, vitamin E 400 mg, and two or three pods of crushed raw garlic in a large spoonful of extra virgin olive oil, first thing in the morning. Very soon, my aunt started feeling much better. Her heart condition improved miraculously, defying the mistaken opinion and the unsound conclusion of her cardiologist. My uncle followed this up with a variety of additional heart-healing essential herbs. My aunt recovered and lived into her eighties in very good health.

Encouraged by this result, I started on large doses of CoQ10, Omega 3 fish oil, crushed raw garlic in a large tablespoon with extra virgin olive oil, and 400 mg of Evion Vitamin E capsules, every day. The rest is history. I was 52 years old when I had my heart attack, and as I write this book today, I am 85 years old and counting, in great health and fine shape. Looking back 30 years later, I remember that Dr Mandke gave me a life expectancy of another 10 years. It has now been 30 years. Many friends tell me I am very lucky to have survived two massive heart attacks in my early fifties. I consider myself not merely lucky, but blessed. I found that if you have the determination and a deep desire to heal yourself, improve, and augment your health, you will live a long, fruitful, and active life, physically, emotionally, and mentally. My purpose in life was to be as happy and contented as possible.

His Holiness Vishwaguru, Swamiji Maheshwaranda, wrote in his book, *Yoga in Daily Life*:

Health is not everything, but everything without health is nothing.

I have a list of 21 medicines that cannot be found in any pharmacy.

1. Laughter is medicine.

2. Loving yourself is medicine.

3. Loving others is medicine.

4. Having good friends is medicine.

5. Good and restful sleep for at least seven to eight hours is medicine.

6. Rays of the early morning sun are medicine.

7. Counting our blessings is medicine.

8. Being grateful is medicine.

9. Forgiving is medicine.

10. Eating correctly and not in excess is medicine.

11. Exercise is medicine.

12. Long walks in nature are medicine.

13. Practising yoga is medicine.

14. Deep conscious breathing is medicine.

15. Meditation is medicine.

16. Drinking plenty of water is medicine.

17. Eating natural foods, fruits, and vegetables is medicine.

18. Occasional fasting is medicine.

19. Letting go of bitter experiences and sorrowful and heart-breaking memories of the past is medicine.

20. Being optimistic in life is medicine.

21. Being enthusiastic, positive, and socially active is medicine.

—— CHAPTER ——
2

SMOKING KILLS, SLOWLY BUT SURELY

How many of us have grown up with the macho Marlboro Man? We longed to emulate the masculine advertising image of the Marlboro Man.

I started smoking because I wanted to look cool and sound cool. "Taking a drag" was oh-so-cool back at age 18 in college. The drag dragged on and soon it had become a habit. An unbreakable habit. In college, I graduated from Charminar to the filtered brand Four Square. I started with three cigarettes a day, one after breakfast, lunch, and dinner. Soon, those three cigarettes a day turned into one pack of 10 cigarettes daily. Like every other smoker, I boasted that I could give up smoking anytime I chose. Famous last words!

Someone once told me the meaning of the word *habit.*

Take away the *H* from *habit* and what remains is *abit—a bit.*

Take away the *A* and *bit* remains. Take away the *B* and *it* still remains. *It* is a habit that is hard to kick. I had become a chain smoker. I would smoke when I was happy. I would smoke when I was not. I would smoke more when I was under stress. Smoking became a part of my everyday life. Cigarettes were an extension of my index and middle finger.

My career with its motto of *breakfast in Bombay, lunch in London, and dinner in New York,* did not help at all. By the time I became an in flight supervisor and manager, I was smoking my all-time favourite brand, Dunhill, and—hold your breath to get away from my smoke—two to three packs of twenties a day. I was like Old Faithful in Yellowstone National Park. Instead of erupting with regularity, smoke curled out of my nostrils every 20 to 30 minutes.

My entire world was trying to make me give up smoking. My wife Maloo and my daughters, Zeena and Jennifer, constantly nagged me. They tormented me to kick the butt, but it was all in vain. How easily we smokers call it nagging and tormenting. When we are under the addictive influence of nicotine, we don't see the love and care that masks their anxiety.

At times, to please my family, I would crumple and crush almost full packs of cigarettes and throw them out of the window saying, "Okay, I give up!" But like a drunk stumbling towards a drink, I would sneak out of the door early the next morning and pick up those badly crumpled packs, straighten out the fire sticks, and try to fix them again to have a smoke. If you asked me to give an arm and a leg, I would do so readily, as long as you keep your grasping hands off my cigarettes.

After some time, love and care become background noise to the main show. You and your nicotine fix.

My elder brother Rusi, living in New York, had a single-point agenda with me. "Hey Noshir, it is enough, more than enough! Get smart and give up smoking! It will kill you. Why should you be the exception?" was his constant lament. When I was posted in London and my routine was to only operate flights between London and New York, Rusi enrolled me in a full course of six private hypnosis sessions, 30 minutes each. Each session cost my brother US$100 per session.

This New York hypnotist tried to mesmerise me into hating the sight of cigarettes. He assured me and my brother that I would loathe the look, the taste, the smoke, and the smell of cigarettes for the rest of my life after six sessions. He had made us believe that he was a magician who would just say, "Whoosh!" and the urge to smoke cigarettes would disappear from my life. But what I found hilarious and got Rusi mad was that towards the end of my sessions, the hypnotist started bumming my British-made Dunhills from me! Physician, heal thyself!

That was US $ 600 down the drain, and I kept thinking, "Boy, I could have bought so many cigarettes with that money."

I continued to smoke in my brother's air-conditioned car. I smoked in their bedroom. I smoked in my bedroom with my daughters in the room. I smoked in the dining room, and everyone complained that the food tasted and smelled like tobacco and nicotine. I had become a nuisance and an unwelcome guest, but I just could not break the smoking habit.

Until the year 1978.

Maloo's legs, ankles, and cheeks were swelling up with water retention. Her creatine levels were sky-high, and her blood pressure hit the roof. After all the tests, my dearest wife was diagnosed with a major kidney problem. The medical name for her condition was Glomerulonephritis, and she was referred to Jaslok Hospital.

The Dean of Jaslok Hospital, Chief Nephrologist and Surgeon, Dr A. S. Mani, was her doctor. And no, I did not make any Noshir-type jokes calling him Dr A. S. Money. The prognosis was a possible kidney replacement. Organ transplants were exceedingly rare at that time. And there was a long queue for kidney transplants.

For the first time in a long while, it felt like the ground beneath my feet was a sinkhole. I was scared, frightened, apprehensive, and very, very nervous. One day, I gave way to my anguish and sobbed loudly, gulping tears, thinking I was alone. I did not notice that my seven-year-old daughter Jennifer had crept up to me. She settled onto my lap and turned around to hold me by my chin. "Noshir Papa, don't cry. I will give Mama my kidneys. No need to wait." She used her baby-sized fists to wipe away my tears. That made me feel even more helpless, and I sobbed, holding her warm, loving body in my arms.

I was the first person in line to donate my kidney. My wife's aunt, Bahia, was trying to jump the queue because Maloo was her favourite niece, and she insisted that her kidney was earmarked for Maloo if required. I'm sure there were other people in the queue, but I was too distraught to notice.

Before people in the queue started to arm wrestle each other, Dr A. S. Mani decided to do one more biopsy of Maloo's kidneys to make the final decision on the kidney transplant. He said there was a one-in-ten chance of an oral cure with a medication regimen. The tests from the biopsy would be checked in the hospital laboratory to see if any combination of drugs could help in curing her diseased kidneys.

When the day for the biopsy rolled around, Maloo checked into Jaslok Hospital. My in-laws, Minoo Papa and

Shirin Mama, and two friends, Ramesh Angle, and Freddy Balsara, were with me, seated outside the operating theatre in Jaslok waiting for the verdict.

Noshir moved away from the worried family members and friends. His constant companion—a red-tipped cigarette—consoled him while tears snaked their way down his gaunt cheeks. He rested his elbows on his knees and dropped his head on his palms, the lit cigarette making it look as if his brain was spewing smoke. It was time for a deal. A deal with the Almighty. What could he use to barter? He had nothing—a loving family did not have any street value. Its emotional quotient was priceless, but its exchange value was zilch.

If Dr Mani were to come out from the operating theatre and put his hands on Noshir's shoulder and say, "Noshir, stop crying. I have good news for you. Your wife will not need a transplant. We can handle this with medications," what would Noshir do? What sacrifice would he make in exchange for that piece of news, that release from agony, that desperate hope of an intact family?

The cigarette forgotten in his moment of angst burned down to the filter, and the untapped ash quivered as if it did not want to drop until a decision had been made. A deal made; a sacrifice promised.

The ash, giving up its fight with gravity, dropped to the floor. Noshir flung the cigarette butt into the ashtray—his mind made up. He would give up smoking then and there. Forever. Was it too late for this sacrifice? Was the Almighty listening?

There was a tap on my shoulder. I jerked up from my reverie, where my mind wandered, and brought myself back to the present—outside the operating theatre in Jaslok Hospital. I looked at Dr A. S. Mani with pleading eyes. "Come to my office," he said. "I have good news." I felt as if a 1000-volt electric shock had shot through my body. I felt the shock physically!

I dropped my cigarette and crushed it under my ankle-high boots. My sacrifice had begun.

I followed Dr A. S. Mani to his office. And the rest, as they say, is history.

That was the last cigarette of my life. The miracle was not that I stopped smoking. The miracle was that, after that moment, I never ever craved a smoke. People warned me about withdrawal symptoms and always sniffed discreetly around me, trying to catch me cheating. They looked at me with disbelief, that giving up my chain-smoking habit was that easy and effortless. Sometimes I couldn't believe it myself. My words to people trying to give up addictive habits would be: You do not need strong willpower to give up the habit. You only need strong motivation. Pick your motivation. In my case, it was my wife's kidney transplant.

As I write the above, I have an icy, chilling feeling creeping up my spine. Within a few seconds after the first puff, noxious chemicals, and the toxic poison in the tobacco smoke reach your heart, lungs, brain, and almost every organ and everywhere your blood goes, damaging your body. Chronic smokers have a very high risk of acquiring a range of potentially very destructive and ultimately devastatingly fatal diseases.

Smoking causes cancer, coronary heart disease, COPD (chronic obstructive pulmonary disease), lung diseases, chronic respiratory conditions, breathing problems, bronchitis, emphysema, tuberculosis, cerebrovascular disease (which damages arteries that supply blood to the brain), and kidney and liver problems. Smoking damages blood vessels, clogs arteries, and much, much more. Need I say more?

People who smoke throughout their lives are prone to cancer of the lungs, throat, oesophagus, larynx, mouth, tongue, nasal passages, stomach, liver, bladder, prostate, pancreas, kidneys, bone marrow, cervix, ureter, and ovaries.

In short, smoking is the main cause (sadly, however preventable) of illnesses and deaths in the world today.

Some smokers claim that they do not inhale the smoke. Not true. Even if they think they do not inhale tobacco smoke, they should know that they still absorb the damaging chemicals through the thin lining of the skin in the mouth. The different chemical contents in tobacco smoke can ravage and cause havoc to your body in many different ways.

So, whichever way you see it, smoking WILL harm your body, slowly but surely.

Here are some of the chemicals:

1. **Nicotine:**

   Nicotine narrows and clogs your arteries and veins. Your heart has to work much harder and faster to distribute the blood to your extremities. It also slows your blood flow, which reduces the oxygen to different organs.

2. **Tar:**

   Tar is a dark brown, very sticky, and smelly jelly-like substance that clogs and coats your lungs.

3. **Carbon monoxide:**

   Carbon monoxide is a poison that binds to haemoglobin in the blood, greatly reducing the ability of the blood to carry oxygen to the various organs in the body, including the brain.

4. **Irritant minute particles:**

   These tiny particles in the tobacco smoke hurt and irritate the throat and lungs, producing mucus and phlegm, causing what we call "a smoker's cough". This is not merely an irritant; it damages the inner throat lining and lungs.

5. **Ammonia:**

   Ammonia is a toxic, colourless, highly irritating, and suffocating gas that hurts the eyes, nasal passages, and throat. Exposure to ammonia in large quantities can be fatal.

6. Tobacco smoke is imbued with cancer-causing chemicals that cause the cells to grow and multiply abnormally at a very rapid pace, turning the cells cancerous.

There are four kinds of smokers:

Beginners:

First-time smokers who start smoking due to peer pressure, curiosity, or just a macho, Marlboro Country style. This stage of smoking is called "getting hooked".

Casual smokers:

Those who smoke two or three cigarettes a day: on waking up, with a cup of coffee, after a meal, with a drink, and/or at party time. This stage is also called "being hooked".

Regular smokers:

This is an advanced stage of smoking when it has become an addictive habit.

Chain smokers:

This sub-group is those who may not need a match or lighter, except for their first cigarette of the day. These smokers light their next cigarette directly with the previously lit cigarette, forming a chain.

Here is a list of different cancers that smokers fall victim to:

1. Breast cancer.

2. Lung and oesophagus cancer.

3. Blood cancer.

4. Stomach and colon cancer.

5. Prostate, bladder, and kidney cancer.

6. Gallbladder, pancreas, and liver cancer.

7. Cervical and uterine cancer.

8. Lymphatic cell cancer.

9. Bone and bone marrow cancer.

This list is only about cancer-related diseases due to smoking. There are many other incurable, more cruel, and frightful diseases that smoking can cause.

After reading this fateful list, if the reader still persists with the smoking habit, it would be nothing short of foolishly suicidal.

On the subject of being suicidal, there is a present-day conflict between the Mental Health Care Act and the Indian Penal Code. The Indian Penal Code experts claim that only suicide attempts caused by extreme and severe stress are not punishable. Smoking does not fall into this category. The act of smoking is an attempt at slow, self-poisoning, amounting to suicide, and is thus punishable under the Indian Penal Code IPC 309, which criminalises the attempt to commit suicide. Smokers beware!

Here is a World Health Organization (WHO) quote about smoking: "Besides being the leading cause of lung cancer, tobacco consumption also multiplies the risk of cancer in the oral regions like mouth, throat, stomach, and urinary bladder."

Another WHO quote: "A single cigarette contains 7,000 chemicals, of which 69 have proven to be carcinogenic."

Need I say more?

Even today, I have friends who are still smokers, who are trying to quit the habit. For them and others trying to quit, I have some suggestions.

1. The internet has a barrage of suggestions that can help, from nicotine patches to hypnosis, from electronic cigarettes to a range of nicotine replacement therapies, such as nasal sprays, mouth sprays, lozenges, willpower, motivation, etc.

2. Read this chapter again. And again. And again. Let it sink in. Set a date to quit. When D-day arrives, read this chapter again. And again. And again. Understand the reasons WHY you need to quit. Motivate yourself. In moments of weakness, when you feel like reaching for a cigarette *just this once*, think of the hundred reasons why you quit. Wait, let the craving pass. It will pass.

But it will come again. Each time, the yearning and longing will be lesser and lesser. Be firm. Be strong. In a few days, the compulsion will diminish to a meagre urge. Soon the urge will pass.

Moreover, smoking not only harms the smoker but harms those around you through second-hand smoke, which can cause similar health issues in non-smokers, particularly children and pregnant women.

The captivating and enslaving nature of nicotine makes quitting quite challenging. However, the rewards of stopping and breaking the habit can instantly, from day one, result in improved health, increased lifespan, and quality of life, which are significantly abundant.

Before you know it, you will be on the road to total freedom.

Your determination to quit may save you from a slow death or a sudden death in the future.

Good luck!

CHAPTER 3

THE POWER OF POSITIVE THINKING

Good thoughts, good words, good deeds—these six words are the basis, premise, doctrine, and foundation of the Zoroastrian religion. My mother also taught me the importance of these words. What you think and what you say is what you are. Your thoughts rule every aspect of your life. You are who you believe you are. What you say to yourself matters the most. Pay attention to self-talk throughout the day. The words we say to ourselves work both ways.

The power of positive thinking is phenomenal. It is euphoric. It has many health benefits. Scientists have been carrying out research on how and why a positive state of mind manifests in good health. A positive outlook can reduce the chances of death from many serious illnesses like heart attack, stroke, and lung infections. It lowers the risk of succumbing to depression. It helps with coping mechanisms when faced with distress, pain, or hardships that are inevitable in life. Positivity leads to better physical and mental health and increases longevity. People also recover from ailments more quickly and adapt better to their everyday life.

People with a positive mindset smile more often and laugh more frequently. The world loves being around them. Both positive and negative thoughts are very powerful but have opposite effects.

A positive person is an optimist. They will always see the bright side in every situation. For them, every grey cloud will have a silver lining. A negative person is a pessimist. They not only dim their own light but also cast dimness and darkness on those around them, affecting their moods and leading to unhappiness, annoyance, and resentment.

An optimist sees their glass half full, while a pessimist sees their glass half empty.

An optimist always looks for the good in every problem and difficulty. Instead of cursing the darkness, they light a candle. Pessimists only focus on what's missing. Constant pessimism wears down and destroys relationships, leaving such people isolated, friendless, and deserted.

Optimists always believe that everything in life will eventually work out and succeed. They say, "Thinking makes it so." Pessimists do not admit or agree that they are pessimists. They often hide under a cloak, saying they are realists. Their negativity makes them believe that everyone is after them and the whole world is gunning for them.

Optimism makes you content, hopeful, healthy, and blessed. It makes you immune to stress. You can always relate to others and make healthy choices. Pessimism impacts your physical and mental health. It also affects your relationships with others in life.

Studies show that positive thinkers tend to be healthier, more sprightly, and more tolerant, and even have a knack for making friends faster than a puppy in a dog park.

Positive thinking enhances your mind, elevates your mood, and can turn even the most humdrum chores into a mini experience.

Remember, a smile and laughter are contagious. So why not spread the laughter and joy and see how many good fellow feelings you can collect.

Imagine waking up each day with a leap, a skip, and a bounce in your step, ready to undertake anything that comes your way.

Positive thinking is like having a trusted umbrella on a rainy day. While the clouds might be looming on the horizon, it keeps you dry and gleeful. Besides, if you are a positive thinker, you will see a silver lining in every cloud you see. If you are a negative thinker, you will only see more rain coming.

You are not just dodging raindrops, you are inviting a whole march-past of options to dance into your life.

So, whether you are sipping your coffee from a half-full cup or a half-empty cup, it is all about your viewpoint and the way you think.

However, on a lighter note, it is said that you should always borrow money from a pessimist. They won't expect it back.

CHAPTER
4

THE BENEFITS OF WALKING

"Fit & Fine at 99 and Beyond?" When it comes to being fit, the first thing that comes to mind is walking. All we need to do is put one foot in front of the other. Do that a couple of thousand times and you reap a hundred health benefits for your body and your soul. A very uncomplicated, elementary exercise with a million benefits. Always remember that the marathon of 26.2 miles begins with the first step.

The simple task of walking is the best gift we can give ourselves. It is a way of exercise we do reflexively every day and has a multitude of health benefits. Besides doing wonders for general health, walking generates happy, feel-good hormones like serotonin, dopamine, endorphin, and oxytocin. Daily walking uplifts your mood, increases your energy levels, and improves your sleep cycle, digestion, and memory. A regular walking schedule can help you much more than merely losing weight. You can prevent many health issues pertaining to your heart, lungs, joints, and muscles. It helps insulin management, controls blood sugar levels, and is good for diabetics. Regular brisk walking improves lung capacity and general stamina. It opens up and clears the blood vessels. As a result, it reduces the risk of heart attacks and strokes. Walking reduces plaque formation in the arteries, veins, and capillaries, which reduces the risk of heart attacks.

Out of the many body-conditioning activities for a healthy lifestyle, daily walking is always on top of the chart. Walking outdoors with nature, early morning or late evening, can be invigorating. It can never be boring, dull, or humdrum. Walking with nature—in a park, a play area, a public garden, or a green lawn—is preferable if possible. A brisk 30 to 45-minute walk about five to six days a week is just what the good doctor ordered. You don't need a personal trainer, heavy equipment, or an expensive gym membership. All you need is a good pair of walking shoes, a bottle of water in hand, your favourite music in your ears, an open walking track, or a green park.

In crowded cities with heavy traffic and limited sidewalks, working out at a gym has become the norm. Yes, gymming, as it is called these days, is very beneficial to the whole body and a great change of lifestyle. Any physical movement of the body is good. Going to the gym is great but not a must. For some, heavy exercises like weightlifting, jogging, and cardio become a punishing routine that gets tedious, monotonous, repetitive, and tiresome. If you lack motivation or do not have the time and inclination to be at the gym every day, make a plan to walk instead as a simple and effective alternative to gymming.

Forget elegant and swanky gyms! Walking is the first original exercise. Just think of it like an elaborate scavenger hunt for fresh air and the random squirrel that is clearly judging your physical fitness level.

Walking can turn your frown into a smile. Who needs therapy when you can take a stroll with Bose headphones and your favourite music in your ears? You can pretend you are part of a music video, Boney M, or doing the moonwalk. Other walkers in the park may think you have lost it. But who cares! Become a trendsetter in the world of "who cares".

Every step is a potential jaunt and an outing.

Who knew your every step could provide entertainment and a diversion for onlookers? And no tickets are required.

Walking stimulates the brain. Suddenly, you are solving life's mysteries, like when you walked into a room and forgot what you needed. It happens all the time.

Walk your way to good health by developing a habit of starting your day early with a brisk morning walk.

Why just walk when you can wave at a friend, dodge a dog, and also trip all at once? It is a workout for both the body and the brain.

So lace up your walking shoes. Embrace and allow your inner dancer, and hit the pavement or a neighbourhood park where every step is an adventure and every stumble is a punchline.

Here are the key benefits of walking daily.

1. Weight management

2. Improved cardiovascular health

3. Lower risks of diseases like diabetes, heart disease, and certain lung diseases

4. Reduced stress and mental well-being

5. Better quality of sleep

6. Increased energy levels

7. Enhanced immune functions

8. Stronger bones and muscles

9. Improved balance and coordination

10. Low-impact form of exercise

11. Release of happiness hormones in the body like dopamine, serotonin, endorphins, and oxytocin, giving you a feel-good factor.

Remember "Fit & Fine at 99 and beyond" is what we all are aiming for.

A wise man once told me that worry does not take away tomorrow's troubles, but it takes away today's peace.

CHAPTER
5

OVERCOME WORRY, STRESS, AND ANXIETY

Worry, stress, and anxiety may be part of life, but they don't have to be the main event.

Always remember that most of the stress comes from the way you react. It is not the path life is. Adopt and modify your viewpoint and all that additional stress will just go away.

Working hard for something we don't care about is called stress.

Working hard for something we love and enjoy is called passion.

With a sprinkle of humour and a touch of silliness, you can challenge those feelings directly—face to face. So go forth, take a deep breath, and remember life is too short to take so seriously. Keep smiling and let the good times roll.

Remember how untroubled and happy-go-lucky you were as a child. Channel that zeal, that same spirit, and get up and go.

Do something stupid, dance in the rain, jump in a puddle. Doing something silly will instantly lift your spirits and show you that life does not have to be taken so seriously.

Watch a funny movie. Watch Charlie Chaplin, Marx Brothers, Laurel and Hardy, and Mr Bean on YouTube. Read a dumb joke book. It has been scientifically proven that laughing reduces stress. Laughter is the best medicine.

Besides, know that it is harder to worry when you are busy reading a joke book.

Feeling anxious, worried, or stressed? Don't stress. (Well, maybe a little, let's keep it light.)

Know you are not alone.

Occasional anxiety is quite normal. It happens before an important interview, a crucial examination, or before delivering a public speech. It is stage fright and may make you momentarily dry in the mouth and maybe even a bit fuzzy.

Continuous stress and worries can provoke anxiety, which can bring about digestive issues like irritable bowel syndrome (IBS) that affect the gastrointestinal tract with abdominal pains, cramping, bloating, gas, diarrhoea, and an upset stomach.

Excessive anxiety can result in depression. Persistent weariness, feelings of sadness, misery, and loss of interest in everyday life are signs of impending depression. Depression is a stealthy burglar that steals your happiness and good cheer, leaving behind melancholy, gloom, and emptiness in its wake. When the underlying feeling of hopelessness becomes all-consuming and interferes with your day-to-day life, it can produce a range of physical, psychological, and emotional issues that are all detrimental to one's general health and peace of mind.

There is undue apprehension and a perpetual fear about familiar everyday situations. There is a feeling of being overwhelmed and of approaching imminent doom and disaster. The physical manifestations of this result in ragged and quick, uneven breathing, shaking, sweating, restlessness, and a pounding, accelerated heart rate.

Adequate sleep, regular physical activity, relaxation techniques like deep breathing and regular meditation, and a well-balanced diet play a significantly crucial role in reducing the effects of stress, anxiety, and depression.

While anxiety is one cause, there is no single cause for depression. It may be triggered by different prompts and reasons. Common reasons are extended illness, death of a loved one, job loss, financial problems, divorce, excessive use of alcohol and/or drugs, and other stressful life events. These multiple scenarios require a multifaceted approach to treating depression.

Sometimes seeking a helping hand and a willing listening ear from close family and friends can provide the required beneficial support. However, it is a good idea (and, in fact, essential) to reach out for qualified professional help from psychologists, psychotherapists, or psychiatrists if the anxiety persists. Besides counselling, and sometimes group counselling, prescription medication, fine-tuned under medical supervision, can work wonders with depression. If left untreated, anxiety, stress, and a depressed state of mind can lead to very serious consequences and are detrimental to the physical and mental health of the person.

A positive mind gives you a much happier and healthier life. It brightens and points the way to limitless possibilities, inner tranquillity, and harmony.

Negativity not only affects the present but also leads and charts your future down dark paths and avenues. It limits your potential and inhibits possibilities for growth. The long-term repercussions of this affect both the person and their interaction with others.

Worrying often just clouds your perception and robs your common sense. Worry devours your energy, preventing you from zeroing in on solutions. Bear in mind that many of the things we worry about may never take place or they are outside your control. Stressing over them is beyond your jurisdiction. Stressing over them doesn't change the outcome. Instead, clutch the present moment. Take proactive steps towards your aspirations and practice gratitude. Remind yourself that you have the strength to handle whatever crosses your path or comes your way.

As is frequently said: *Laugh and the world laughs with you. Cry and you cry alone.* There is no need to cry alone with so many remedies at your fingertips.

Anger and rage are violent emotions that can unsettle lives if uncontrolled. Timely and effective anger management can transform this kind of hostility into inner peace.

CHAPTER
6

ANGER AND ANGER MANAGEMENT

Managing anger can sometimes feel like trying to tame a wild beast. But with a sprinkle of creativity and a dash of humour, it can become a lot more manageable.

We all experience anger off and on. It often feels like an excuse for an emotional outlet, a kind of release. But one must control one's anger and not the other way around. If anger controls you, it becomes your master, and you, its slave. Anger does not solve anything. It only destroys everything. It is the fire that scorches the hand that holds it.

Anger comes from a variety of sources and for different reasons. Personal unsolvable problems. Stressful situations. The intensity of anger varies depending on the person and the situation. While it is quite normal to feel angry upon provocation, getting angry in situations beyond your control is futile. It can hurt and damage both physical and emotional health. Anger is a very heavy load to bear: it burdens the heart, soul, and spirit, leaving no room for peace and happiness.

Recurrent and uncontrolled rage turns to animosity and fury. This increases blood pressure, accelerates heart rate, and increases the release of cortisol, the stress hormone. Uncontrolled anger is self-destructive. It feeds on itself, ruining all relationships. Hurting loved ones ends up with both sides making impulsive, unjustified, and outrageous decisions. Anger brings about emotional upheaval, causes irreparable damage, and creates physical distance from the closest of loved ones. Intense exasperation leads to physical and verbal abuse and terminates good relationships. It brings about negative repercussions in one's life, breaking long-term kinship.

Extreme anger can often lead to agony and trauma. It is a chain that fastens around us and constricts us, ensnaring us in a cycle of apathy and mayhem. Long-drawn-out anger has negative effects on mental well-being, gives rise to cardiovascular complications, results in a poor immune system, and many other health issues. Chronic short temper, often referred to as having a very short fuse, has various harmful effects on the body, including conditions like chronic digestive issues such as IBS, and can also impact mental health leading to depression and anxiety. Sometimes anger is so deeply rooted and entrenched in the heart and mind of the person that it kills the spirit of the human being inside.

Anger clouds the mind. It misrepresents and distorts vision and leads to actions you will regret later. The results of anger are more painful than the reasons for anger. Holding on to anger is like taking in poison and expecting the other individual to die.

I had a friend named Aslam Ali who is now no more. He and his brother developed an enmity beyond sanity, beyond comprehension. They had so much anger, hatred, and animosity towards each other that it was deranged and outrageous. Aslam Ali once told me that when he died, he didn't know if he wanted to go to heaven or hell. I told him it wasn't in our hands but asked which one he would prefer (Stupid question!). He said if his brother had gone to heaven, he would prefer to go to hell. I was shocked by this anger and hatred that carried on into the afterlife. So much hostility! So much resentment! It was hard for me to digest this much bad blood between two blood brothers.

How do we contain and manage our temper, anger turning into rage, rage into wrath, and finally exploding out of control?

Anger management is an art. If practised regularly, it can create long-term peace and tranquillity in the body and mind. Addressing and managing anger through healthy adaptation strategies is very essential for general happiness and wellness. Handling any and all situations to manage anger is the best thing you can do for yourself. Managing anger is one of the most important virtues one can practice.

There are a few basic and fundamental steps to follow and believe in:

1. **Practice deep breathing:**

   When angry, take slow, deep breaths through the nose and hold. Blow out and exhale very slowly through the mouth. Do this several times until you calm down and your anger subsides.

2. **Recognise the cause:**

   Recognise the triggers that make you angry. Identify the situation, the scenario that started it, and the people who aggravated the situation. Awareness is the first step in managing the upcoming anger before it becomes ongoing anger.

3. **Take a break:**

   Give yourself a moment. Count to 10 slowly. Give yourself some time and space to compose yourself. Relax, get a grip, and cool down.

4. **Remove yourself:**

   Remove yourself temporarily from the situation, if possible. This will give you a breather to regain your serenity and composure to calm down.

5. **Communicate:**

   Communicate calmly, yet firmly, without any confrontation or hostility. Express your feelings clearly without condemning anybody.

6. **Inject humour:**

   Find ways to infuse a bit of humour. Light-hearted jocularity can be a very helpful strategy to shift the focus and diffuse the intensity from escalating into anger. Humour creates a more favourable atmosphere.

7. **Seek professional help:**

   If you still find it challenging to cope, seeking professional help would be a wise decision. A counsellor or a therapist can provide further guidance and show you various strategies and resources to curb your anger.

Breaking free from anger makes you a happier and healthier person, both physically and emotionally.

Remember, anger is a normal emotion. But also know that frequent and explosive anger will hurt you more than the person you are angry with.

You think you are punishing them, but you are actually left with a bad case of regret or a no-return situation.

It is like throwing a boomerang. You might aim at someone else. But guess who is going to get hurt, right between the eyes? Yourself.

Controlling a beast, whether literal or metaphorical, is, as I said earlier, a mix of composure, tenacity, understanding, and the right approach. If all fails, try humour.

Just like a wild animal, awareness of what provokes your beast is the key. Determining the reason can help you tackle it more successfully.

Undertake the situation with calmness. Yelling at a beast usually only makes it more violent and ruthless. Try using a calming and comforting voice. Try using humour in the situation, and you will disarm your anger before it has a chance to roar.

Just like a beast needs a den, you too need a sanctuary to cool down. Find a cosy spot where you too can retreat to cool off and gather your thoughts before re-entering the fray.

The key to a joyful long life is embracing happiness daily.
Always remember, a smile is a spiritual perfume you
spray on others.

CHAPTER
7

LOVE, LIVE, LAUGH AND LONGEVITY

Living life king-size means adding life to your years, not years to your life. Living life large is about savouring life's essences and making each day a royal feast of life's possibilities and opportunities.

Enfolding love, laughter, and gusto for life can substantially upgrade and enrich our wellness and longevity. Love promotes strong social and family ties, which are vital for psychological and emotional health and can minimise anxiety.

Laughter initiates the release of endorphins, elevating the immune system and promoting calmness of the mind and body. Living fully by courting passions and ambitions, fostering relationships, and maintaining a positive outlook on life contribute to overall happiness and adaptability.

Together, these components create a very fulfilling life, curtailing the effects of ageing and promoting a healthier and longer life expectancy.

The human body is complex but is designed to last for an average lifespan of 70 to 80 years. Beyond that is a rare bonus. So let us all hold tight and embrace each moment with meaningful living and memories.

Live every moment with grandeur, pursue your passions boldly, and discover magnificence in all your experiences.

The body undergoes a natural ageing process. Over time, organs begin to decline in their functioning abilities. Body cells and body tissues begin a slow death. However, one can slow down and delay the process of ageing by keeping the body cells, body tissues, and organs healthy longer by adopting certain lifestyle changes. The secret of long life involves a combination of factors that are dependent on the individual.

Living a long, healthy life is a goal for some and a dream for many. That goal requires much more than merely avoiding illnesses. It is about incorporating an all-round holistic approach to life that results in better well-being and longevity.

Here is a small list of essential keys to unlock a healthier mind and body for a longer life.

Regular physical activities like walking, strength training, cardio, flexibility, and yoga.

A well-balanced nutritional diet. Focus on fruits, multicoloured vegetables, lean proteins, seafood, healthy fats, and grains.

Practice a routine of quality sleep. Aim for restful REM, core, and seven to eight hours of deep, undisturbed sleep. Try to maintain a consistent sleep schedule. Ensure that your bedroom is cool and dark to provide a restful environment. Consider reading under a bedside lamp before falling asleep.

Avoid all forms of tobacco consumption and smoking that harm your health and are proven to shorten one's lifespan. Drink alcohol in moderation or avoid it altogether.

Be aware of your mental health and wellness. Stay away from people who make you anxious and/or depress you.

Stave off loneliness by maintaining strong ties socially. Have a close circle of supportive friends and participate in community activities.

Never stop learning. Engage in activities that challenge your mind, like Crossword puzzles, Word search and Sudoku, that task your mind. Involve yourself in forms of creativity that you enjoy.

Make sure you take annual or semi-annual health check-ups. Be an advocate for your health by taking the initiative and being proactive. Preventive healthcare is a more economical alternative than ending up in the emergency room with a critical health issue. Catch the disease early.

Have a positive outlook. Positivity increases one's longevity. Find reasons for laughter and joy in your life. Practice gratitude and be optimistic in all situations in your life.

I would categorise six moral principles for a happy life:

1. Listen before you speak.

2. Think before you write.

3. Earn before you spend.

4. Try before you give up.

5. Believe before you pray.

6. Live before you die.

When we talk about longevity, Japanese, Scandinavians, and Icelanders come to mind. Several components contribute to their longer lifespans.

1. **Healthy diet:**

   Their traditional cuisine includes a variety of nutritionally healthy and fresh seasonal foods, such as seafood, fresh fruits and vegetables, minimal oil, grains, rice, and tofu. This is very heart-healthy and heart-friendly.

2. **Excellent healthcare system:**

The Japanese public has easy access to a well-developed healthcare system. The country has a very efficient and easily available support system and health benefits, including vaccination campaigns, health education, and advanced preventive healthcare services.

3. **Low rate of obesity:**

Maintaining a normal weight is often linked to a lower rate of health issues. Almost every Japanese and Scandinavian is health-conscious and remains as fit as possible. Compared to other developed countries, Japan and some Northern countries have a much lower rate of obesity.

4. **Excellent healthcare habits:**

The Japanese people engage in regular physical activities like walking, stretching, cardiovascular exercise, gardening, and other tasks which they see as a pleasure. Their active lifestyle contributes to their overall well-being and better health.

5. **Public health initiatives:**

Strong social and community support and a sense of belonging bring about better mental and physical health and a much richer quality of life for the aged.

6. **Genetic factors:**

Good lifestyle habits are passed on from one generation to the next, which contributes to longevity. The Japanese people seldom retire.

Besides Japan, author and explorer Dan Buettner has identified several other regions in the world where many different communities have unusually long and healthy lifespans compared to the rest of the world.

These regions have been identified as blue zones. Okinawa (Japan), Loma Linda (USA), Sardinia (Italy), and Ikaria (Greece) are blue zones. They share common cultural practices, and more or less common diets rich in whole grains, vegetables, fruits, large quantities of fish, and lean protein. They avoid sugar and processed foods. This overall lifestyle contributes to their good health and longevity.

If these blue zones can do it, so can we. Life is a journey. And the path can be as beautiful as you choose to make it.

*Moderate alcohol consumption has some health benefits
and enhances social experiences. However, excessive and
uncontrolled drinking can lead to addiction, liver damage,
and many other health problems.*

CHAPTER

8

CHEERS!! THE GOOD, THE BAD, AND THE UGLY OF ALCOHOL

The one thing that makes passengers groan over international travel is the unearthly hour that they have to arrive at the airport for check-in. It is the same for the crew members. But the passengers see the crew members walking together towards the departure gate, all spruced up and spiffy in their airline uniforms, and are very impressed and satisfied that they are in safe hands. If only! If only!

At all layover stations across Air India's network, crew members check into five-star hotels and supposedly get a good night's rest before the next flight. It was normal practice for the hotel reception desk or telephone operator to give a courtesy wake-up call to each crew member, an hour prior to the pickup time.

At one of these stopovers, we had all checked into the Ashoka Hotel in New Delhi. The wake-up call was at 3:00 am, and the pickup was at 4:00 am for the crew of flight AI 101 from Delhi to London. I was the inflight supervisor for this flight.

By 3:45 am, most of the crew had gathered in the lobby to check out. We were drinking our coffee or tea and preparing to board the bus for the airport. All except Flight Purser Rajoo Mehta. At 3:50 am, I asked the person at the reception desk to give him a reminder call and tell him that the crew were waiting for him in the lobby. The receptionist tried a couple of times, but there was no answer. We thought he must be on his way down.

The lift door pinged, and I turned to give Rajoo Mehta an earful. Out came Rajoo Mehta in all his glory. He was dressed in the covering that nature gave him. Naked as a newborn! Or to be more precise—buck naked! Not completely, though; he had the Air India uniform cap on his head, and his shoes were on his feet, but no socks. He was dishevelled, obviously from imbibing one too many into the wee hours of the morning. He wasn't even like Adam, trying to cover himself with a fig leaf. He carried his briefcase in one hand and his room key in the other, which hung from a heavy and bulky brass plate with the room number attached. He stumbled towards the reception desk to surrender his room key. The young ladies on duty delicately averted their eyes.

Now, there was nothing about Rajoo that would make the damsels avert their eyes when he was fully clothed. He was sweet, pleasantly plump, and an adorable, simple young man. For the young ladies, he was their soft toy, a teddy bear with chubby cheeks.

There was complete silence in the lobby and everyone's gaze fastened on him. Soon, there were some muffled gasps and stifled guffaws. Along with three other crew members, I jumped towards him, and we formed a cordon around him. With Rajoo in the centre, we shuffled like penguins towards the lift doors, and got him in and into his room in quick time.

I had to think fast on my feet to avert an incident. I instructed two of the crew members to go down and instruct the crew waiting downstairs to board the bus and leave for the airport. I told one crew member, Abhishek Kapoor, to stay with me. I called the lobby manager and requested him to arrange a taxi in 10 minutes to take the rest of us to the airport.

And then we got to work on Rajoo. We quickly splashed iced water from the fridge on Rajoo's face. The lobby manager and a lobby assistant raced up to the room to help us get Rajoo moving. They suggested dunking Rajoo's head in ice-cold water. We followed their suggestion. Abhishek Kapoor made some hot black coffee in the room's hotpot and forced Rajoo to drink it.

When he recovered a bit from his stupor, I told Rajoo to report sick and sleep it off. But he fell at my feet, begging me to take him with us on the flight. He did not wish to report sick. He believed that if he did not board the flight, he would probably lose his job. Fortunately, his non-ironed shirt and tie, his uniform jacket, and trousers were hanging in the coat compartment of the room. In 15 minutes, we had shaken him up, dressed him, and brought him down to the lobby again. His bags were already in the lobby, waiting to be identified.

Abhishek Kapoor, Rajoo Mehta, and I jumped into the taxi and told the driver to race to the airport. We reached the airport 25 minutes late. I spoke to the commander about the unfortunate incident at the Ashoka Hotel. I know both of us wanted to clutch each other and collapse into gales of laughter. The commander controlled himself and told me very solemnly that I would have to take full responsibility for Rajoo's behaviour if I wanted him to be on board. And I was also responsible for seeing that Rajoo remained fully dressed throughout the flight. He could not afford to put the reputation of Air India at stake by releasing a flasher among his respectable passengers. I bit down hard on my lips to stop the mirth from spilling out and accepted the challenge.

Cheers!!! is such a euphoric and carefree word. It brings joy, good health, and salutations to everyone who raises his or her glass to celebrate and propose a toast. It holds a collective, cultural, and social significance. It is the war cry for celebrations to begin.

But as a universal announcement of goodwill, it has several different meanings.

1. **Wishing well:**

   When we clink glasses and say, "Cheers," it is a way of wishing each other happiness. It boasts a sense of camaraderie and unity, sharing moments of merriment, high spirits, and like-minded people.

2. **Celebration and jubilation:**

   "Cheers" is often used at festive and celebratory times. By raising a toast, you present and accept the special moment in the present with everybody around you, whether it's a wedding, an engagement, a birth, a birthday, a promotion, a farewell party, or simply an opportunity to enjoy the wonderful company you are in. "Cheers" brings good cheer to the occasion.

3. **Communal spirit:**

   Besides the clinking of glasses and calling a toast, it is a social ritual that envelops shared joy and brings on a communal spirit. It adds a touch of warmth and fondness to the celebration.

Alcohol is usually served at social gatherings, parties, and other celebrations. Partaking in an occasional serving of alcohol at these celebrations is a good thing. Some people who are shy and nervous will loosen up when they come forward.

Moderate consumption is relaxing and helps in social bonding. After a drink or two, even an introvert unwinds and moves into his/her comfort zone with ease. Some studies have shown that moderate alcohol lengthens one's lifespan. It is beneficial to the cardiovascular system and reduces the risk of heart disease. Alcohol is beneficial to the good cholesterol levels and also prevents blood clotting.

The keywords here are caution and moderation. One should never become overly dependent on drinking and addicted to alcohol.

Chronic dependence on alcohol creates an increasing urge to consume larger quantities, more frequently to achieve the same effect on the body and brain. It affects one's mental and physical health in an adverse way. One quickly descends into the dark world of addiction.

Psychologically, one turns to alcohol as a coping mechanism and a tool to handle stress and overcome anxiety. This leads to a constant emotional need for alcohol. By then, it will be too late.

Uncontrolled habitual use of alcohol results in serious liver diseases, such as fatty liver and cirrhosis of the liver. Cirrhosis is mostly irreversible.

Addiction to alcohol usually leads to a one-way street, downhill. There is professional help for alcoholics, including support groups, counselling, and extensive medical help from professionals in the field.

However, on a lighter note, here are some funny toasts you can use for various occasions.

1. **To the married couple:**

   Just remember, a happy marriage is like a deck of cards: In the beginning, all you need is two Hearts and a Diamond. By the end, you are looking for a Club and a Spade.

2. **To ageing:**

   "Here's to ageing! May we grow old gracefully... or at least with a good sense of humour and a well-stocked bar!"

3. **To life:**

   "Here's to life! May it be filled with love, laughter, and just enough bad decisions to keep things interesting!"

4. **To age gracefully:**

   "Here's to ageing gracefully! If we can't be young and beautiful, let us be old and hilarious!"

5. **To health:**

   "Here's to our health, may we stay fit enough to enjoy life and flexible enough to get up from the couch after a TV binge."

6. **To happiness:**

   Here's to happiness!

   May we never forget that a little laughter can add years to our life and a lot of cake can add many inches to our waist!

Raise your glasses and enjoy the laughter.

Remember, humour can be a great way to address serious topics. However, it is important to approach sensitive subjects with care.

Drug addiction can take hold and possess the individual without warning, transforming and making far-reaching changes in lives and relationships to reach a rock-bottom abyss.

CHAPTER

9

DRUGS AND SUBSTANCE ABUSE

Here is a terrifying, very serious, and impactful narration about the horrors of drug use and their potential dangers.

Very sadly, what often begins as a curiosity or a means of escape temporarily very quickly spirals into a living nightmare.

Promoting awareness and prevention is crucial.

The horrors of drug use are a stark reality that is not easy to comprehend, and that many face every day.

Experimenting with drugs at a young age can lead to addiction and severe health issues, and can have devastating consequences on life. It quickly spirals into a nightmare. Drugs can distort our reality, alter our perception, and lead to devastating consequences.

Drugs can enslave you. Once a person becomes dependent, the struggle to break free is almost insurmountable, often leading to a cycle of despair that not only affects the individual but their loved ones as well.

The impact of drugs on individuals and the community can be devastating, leading to major health issues, addiction, and often tragic consequences. Socially, the repercussions are profound. Relationships with friends and family often deteriorate as isolation sets in and trust erodes. Individuals will find themselves alienated from their support network, leading to further emotional setbacks.

Drugs like heroin, marijuana, LSD, hashish, and cocaine are substances that debilitate the body and mutate the mind when consumed. Different drugs have different strange, surreal, weird, and abnormal reactions and after-effects. They produce conflicting feelings of intoxication, rapture, amplified merriment, relaxation, and heightened energy. This leads to crazed mania, derangement, and/or passivity, inactivity, and lethargy. The person is sometimes out for the count in a comatose state, blacks out, and is dead to the world. Certain legal prescription medicines also have the same effect.

Over time, these drugs have very damaging social and economic consequences and cause mental damage affecting long-term health.

Being caught in a drug habit can and will lead to devastating consequences that can permeate every aspect of an individual's life. The body and mind become increasingly dependent on the substance, leading to withdrawal symptoms that can be life-threatening and extremely painful, to say the least.

Financially, the high cost associated with maintaining the drug habit can lead to bankruptcy, hopelessness, homelessness, and legal troubles.

Beyond deteriorating physical health, the psychological toll is even more alarming. Addiction often breeds depression, anxiety, and a very distorted sense of reality, making it impossible for individuals to function properly in their day-to-day lives.

Ultimately, the end results of being caught in a drug habit can be tragic. A cycle of despair where personal dreams are shattered, lives are lost, and potential is wasted, either through overdose or the consequences of a different lifestyle that prioritises drug use over happiness, health, and human connections.

Like excessive usage of alcohol, uninhibited use of drugs leads to addiction, and the person craves increased amounts of the same drug to achieve the same desired exclusionary effect.

This is when the body is subjected to substance abuse and becomes dependent on the daily fix. The brain seeks the drug constantly despite ruinous after-effects. Eventually, there is a danger of frequent overdosing, becoming lethal.

Youngsters fall prey to drugs due to different reasons. Initially, they are attracted to drugs for the exhilaration and anticipation of the unknown surrounding it. They seek drugs for kicks and experimentation as a sense of adventure. Sometimes they could be drawn to it because of peer pressure and see it as a way to fit in and be cool. They seek approval from their peers and want to be welcomed into the elite club of cool dudes. Some of them are drawn to mild drugs as a way to cope with anxiety, stress, mild depression, and emotional needs to meet life's challenges.

Social and cultural factors often glamorise and popularise drug culture through multimedia and word of mouth. Lack of awareness of the hazards and perils of drug use leaves them vulnerable. Easy accessibility of drugs makes it possible to try them out for the first time, then occasionally, and finally get hooked to them. Unfortunately, the vicious cycle and life's downturn start from there. Sadly, it becomes a path of no return.

Drug use is influenced by environmental, psychological, biological, and sociological factors. Prevention efforts should focus on coping skills with various strategies for young people. This includes fostering healthy relationships with children in their teens and providing education and support. Dealing with the situation, being aware of positive alternatives, and developing amicable strategies help teenagers who are ambivalent about the harmful effects of drug usage.

It is the responsibility of elders and society to generate positive opportunities for youth to blossom into maturity and develop as good citizens, taking the road as far away from drugs as possible.

Say "NO" to drugs!

Blood pressure - the silent killer strikes without any outward warning. It silently damages your heart and your blood vessels. Resistant hypertension is lethal.

CHAPTER
10

BLOOD PRESSURE – THE SILENT KILLER

"Blood pressure is a silent killer" is a very common phrase because high blood pressure (hypertension) has no visible indications or symptoms. Hypertension is asymptomatic. This means many people who have it do not know about it until it leads to other medical ramifications. High blood pressure can go undetected for years. This leads to highly dangerous situations with serious health complications if left untreated.

Undetected high blood pressure can lead to life-threatening complications without any warning. Most people are unaware that their blood pressure is elevated, allowing the condition to advance unchecked. Over time, high blood pressure ruins and damages blood vessels and many vital organs, increasing the threat of serious health outcomes such as stroke, kidney failure, and lethal heart disease.

The aggregate and cumulative effects can be disastrous. A sudden heart attack or stroke can strike without any symptoms, leading to irreversible impairment or death. The muffled side effects are varied and can substantially impact the quality of life. Common symptoms can include headaches, dizziness, and fatigue. However, many people may not suffer from any symptoms, which can deprive them of suitable medical care.

Chronic hypertension may lead to complications such as heart failure, kidney failure, diabetes, cognitive decline, and even vision loss. Despite the absence of symptoms, blood pressure does not soar but creeps. High blood pressure develops gradually over time due to various reasons. It could be hereditary or due to lifestyle factors such as smoking, unhealthy diet, consuming salty snacks and foods, or consuming excessive alcohol. Other factors that contribute to it are long-term stress, lack of exercise, being overweight, and living a sedentary lifestyle.

Over time, high blood pressure silently damages the heart, the blood vessels throughout the body, the kidneys, the liver, and other organs in the body. Due to its silent nature, uncontrolled hypertension poses a very high-risk factor for cardiovascular disease and many other life-threatening conditions. Constricting arteries and calcification of the veins (atherosclerosis), weakened and unusually enlarged or thinning of the blood vessels (aneurysms), and other complications become more prevalent with age.

It is a good idea to keep a digital blood pressure machine at home and monitor one's blood pressure routinely. This is a handy machine and it is very convenient to monitor blood pressure for all adults and elders in the family, especially if high blood pressure is detected at a doctor's clinic.

In a doctor's office or clinic, blood pressure sometimes shows an elevated reading when compared to blood pressure taken at home in a relaxed setting. This temporary rise in blood pressure is due to nervousness, stress, and anxiety when one is in a clinical setting and interacting with medical professionals in white coats. It is called white coat hypertension or white coat syndrome. It is estimated that 25 to 30% of people in the world suffer from white coat hypertension.

For doctors to evaluate the true blood pressure readings of such patients, an ambulatory blood pressure monitoring (ABPM) machine is attached to the arm of the patient for a 24-hour period to take readings automatically every 30 minutes.

Another blood pressure-related problem, which is much more acute and grave, is called "Resistant Hypertension." This is a very complex hypertension problem that is not easily controlled and may need six or more different blood pressure medicines taken four to five times a day (almost every two hours) to keep it in reasonable check.

In addition to that, one may have postural hypotension like me, which drops substantially, ending up from very high to very low blood pressure, accompanied by all-consuming, intense dizziness. When one stands up from a sitting or lying position, it gets even more difficult and complicated to keep the blood pressure in decent control, needing very specialised doctors in the field.

I say this from personal experience since I used to suffer from Resistant Hypertension. My blood pressure reading stayed around 200+ over 100+, despite the many different medications that I took every day, every couple of hours.

My daughters, Jennifer and Zeena, had taken me to see Dr Naresh Trahan, Head Cardiologist, Head Surgeon, and Director of Medanta Hospital in Delhi, and cardiac surgeon Dr Mittal, also at Medanta Hospital in Delhi. They are among some of the very best cardiologists and cardiac surgeons in India.

In Mumbai, I was being treated by Dr Ashwin B. Mehta, who has the reputation of being a great interventional cardiologist in Bombay, specialising in controlling erratic blood pressures like mine. After meeting and spending hours with all these experts, I felt confident to place myself in their hands.

However, within a short period of time, my BP again started rocketing sky-high. But with major medication, it would fall to rock bottom, often resulting in sudden dangerous falls.

Another wonderful, kind, and competent doctor is Dr Sushant Daware, head of the ICU at Bombay Hospital. He is a friend and more than family to us. He has been available and looking after us 24/7.

However, despite the best cardiologists' efforts, my body would soon become used to almost all the prescribed medicines, and my BP would once again continue to go all over the place, endangering my life, with a constant fear of an impending stroke or heart failure.

At this stage, my daughter Jennifer spent all her days reading, searching, and researching, trying to find a way to beat my blood pressure.

At last, she discovered a surgeon at the University Hospital in Basel, Switzerland, who is a pioneer in discovering a long-term permanent cure approved by the FDA in the USA for this kind of hypertension. This very latest new-age procedure is known as "Renal Denervation", which burns the nerves around both the kidneys and places stents in the renal arteries for easy blood flow.

My daughter managed to get an appointment for my surgery in Switzerland under Dr Felix Mahafoud. This surgery was nothing short of a miracle for my family and me.

I am happy to add that my "Postural and Resistant Hypertension" is not postural nor resistant anymore. Thanks to the healing hand of Dr Felix Mahafoud and his team, I am good, I am cured.

Blood pressure, what is that?

The insidious nature of high blood pressure underscores the importance of regular health check-ups, as early detection and management can improve overall well-being and prevent severe outcomes.

Thanks to Dr Felix Mahafoud and my family. At this time, "Fit for life," is not a dream at all but a very likely possibility for my wife Maloo and me.

Amen!

Diabetes is like having a complicated relationship with the sweetness of sugar.

It is sweet, very sweet, but cannot and should not be trusted.

CHAPTER

11

HOW TO KEEP DIABETES UNDER CONTROL

Diabetes is a complicated condition that can develop at any age due to a variety of reasons: lifestyle, heredity, and environment.

There are two types of diabetes: Type 1 and type 2.

Type 1 diabetes is generally diagnosed in early childhood. It can also manifest in youngsters. The exact cause of type 1 diabetes is not known. It could be because of genetic factors, certain toxins, or certain viral infections. People with type 1 diabetes need lifelong treatment as the pancreas does not produce adequate insulin to manage the sugar levels in the body.

Type 2 diabetes poses significant hazards to health, impacting various bodily systems and increasing the risk of serious complications. One of the primary dangers is high blood sugar levels, which can lead to nerve damage (Neuropathy), kidney damage (Nephropathy), and vision problems, including diabetic Retinopathy, which can lead to blindness.

One of the other main dangers is the cardiovascular issues. People with diabetes are three to four times more likely to experience a stroke or develop heart disease.

The condition also increases the risk of serious infections, slowing down the healing process of wounds, which often leads to amputation of lower limbs in extreme cases.

Effective control of diabetes often begins with lifestyle changes and major modifications, including adopting a balanced diet rich in lean proteins, vegetables, whole grains, and certain fruits, and drastically reducing sugars and processed foods.

Regular exercises like walking, swimming, outdoor games, etc., aiming for at least 150 minutes of physical activities per week can improve insulin sensitivities and greatly help to control blood sugar levels.

Of course, in many cases, medication may be necessary to help maintain steady glucose levels in the system. Education about the disease and regular monitoring of blood sugar through routine check-ups are all very essential in empowering individuals to take charge of their health and prevent complications from type 2 diabetes cannot be overestimated.

Type 2 diabetes is generally due to hereditary factors, a sedentary lifestyle, physical inactivity, inappropriate diet, and obesity. It also occurs due to advancing age and high blood pressure. Type 2 diabetes mostly impacts adults. The treatment requires different medications, daily insulin shots, exercise, daily walks, and a diet with minimal or preferably zero sugar to control blood sugar levels. The diabetic needs to make some changes in his/her lifestyle such as regular health check-ups, weight loss, diet control, and adopting a beneficial lifestyle.

My wife, Meherangiz N. Sanjana (Maloo), who is 84 years old, has had type 2 diabetes for the last 40+ years. Diabetes is quite rampant in her family. She was on insulin injections four times a day, in addition to allopathic medications twice a day. Despite these medications and injections, her sugar levels fluctuated wildly.

It was then that I started reading about herbal, natural, and traditional Indian remedies available in Ayurveda that are trusted to control sugar levels and promote overall health. She tried different herbal and Ayurvedic remedies that brought down her sugar levels substantially. In fact, I would say "drastically." The sugar readings dipped so low that she cut down on insulin injections from four to only two a day. Seeing her low sugar level readings, her doctor reduced the strength and dosage of her allopathic medicines too.

Here are some Ayurveda herbs that continue to keep her sugar levels down:

1. **Fenugreek seeds (Methi):**

   Soak a large spoonful of methi seeds in half a glass of water overnight. Drink the water, and chew and swallow the methi seeds, first thing in the morning. Methi carries particular compounds and fibre that improve insulin sensitivity and lower sugar levels.

2. **Okra (Lady's fingers or Bhendi in Hindi):**

   Cut and slice four or five okras. Soak them overnight in a glass of water, stir the water, and drink it in the afternoon before lunch.

3. **Bitter gourd (Karela):**

   Karela is another very popular Ayurvedic remedy for diabetes. One karela is blended in a juicer-mixer and served in the evening.

4. **Indian Gooseberry (Amla):**

   Amla is a very potent antioxidant-rich fruit used in Ayurvedic medicine for diabetes management. One or two Amlas after dinner will regulate your sugar.

5. **Turmeric (Haldi):**

   Haldi is a yellow, peppy spice that improves the propensity for insulin, reduces inflammation, and supports overall healthy balance, including diabetes.

6. **Holy Basil (Tulsi):**

   Hallowed in Ayurveda for its medicinal properties, tulsi reduces stress and helps regulate blood sugar.

7. **Indian blackberry or black plum (Jamun):**

   Jamun has tremendous potential to bring the sugar level down. Jamun seeds are crushed into powder and sold in capsule form.

8. Chia seeds, fenugreek seeds, and sliced okra need to be soaked in half a glass of water separately and taken the next day at intervals to keep the sugar levels well under control.

However, the above should not be replaced with other medicines prescribed by your diabetologist. These Ayurveda herbs and prescribed medications should not be taken simultaneously; otherwise, the sugar levels may crash drastically low and prove to be dangerous. Herbal supplements should be used as part of integrated diabetic care and as an add-on to prescribed medication.

Inform your healthcare provider about the additional herbal supplements or remedies you are using so that the allopathic diabetic medication can be fine-tuned.

My wife's diabetes has been well under control for decades now with the help of Ayurveda remedies. It has decreased the need to take higher doses of allopathic medicines as well as the number of insulin injections.

God has been overly kind to us. It is said that God helps the sailor. But the sailor must also row. My wife and I need to thank our very able and beautiful Diabetologist, Dr. Piya Thakkar of Bombay Hospital, who has kept my wife's sugar-levels safe and controlled, all these years.

The kidneys, liver, and pancreas are essential organs that regulate metabolism, maintain sugar levels, and detoxify the body, ensuring overall health and balance.

CHAPTER 12

THE 3 MUSKETEERS: KIDNEY, LIVER, PANCREAS

All for one, and one for all.

Your kidneys, liver, and pancreas play a very significant and crucial role in your overall physical wellness and health. Take utmost care of these three pivotal organs and keep them in top shape.

Liver:

While the largest external organ in our body is the skin, the most voluminous internal organ is the liver. It is located just under the diaphragm in the upper right part of the abdomen.

One of the key functions of the liver involves the production of bile which helps with digestion. It plays an essential role in the metabolism and purification of nourishment from food. The liver intermixes fats for good assimilation in the body. It plays a role in the immune function, hormone regulation, and assimilation of cholesterol.

The liver helps with blood clotting and wound recuperation. It is a storehouse for vitamins and minerals and holds a stockpile of vitamins A, D, and B12, and the body's most important energy source, glycogen.

Another important function of the liver is to detoxify all harmful substances, such as drugs, alcohol, and other waste products by breaking them down and converting them into less toxic compounds for final elimination from the body.

Life depends on the liver.

Kidneys:

Kidneys are bean-shaped organs located on both sides of the spinal column, below the ribs. Our kidneys are very essential organs, and there are a hundred reasons why we must keep them healthy and functioning. The kidneys produce many different hormones in our body that have different functions.

Kidneys manage the blood pressure in our bodies by producing renin that regulates the narrowing and dilating of blood vessels. They activate the bone marrow filled with red blood cells. The kidneys maintain the body's acid-base balance that governs the pH balance of the body fluids, including the blood. This is most important for metabolism and cellular function.

Kidneys also control the sodium and water balance in our system. They produce calcitriol, which activates vitamin D to regulate phosphate and calcium levels in the body.

The kidneys are the body's filtration system. They remove toxins and work as a waste-cleaning system by extracting all waste matter through the urine, thereby obviating the buildup of harmful substances in the body.

It is crucial to keep our kidneys working in optimum condition by getting regular renal function tests done via a simple blood and urine test. Smoking, any form of tobacco ingestion, and/or excessive alcohol consumption damage your kidneys and increase the risk of kidney disease.

Get your blood pressure and sugar levels checked regularly.

Be disciplined in taking any prescribed medications diligently.

Drink plenty of water to stay well hydrated. Don't wait to get thirsty. Drink a bit all the time at short intervals. Research shows that many elderly people do not feel thirsty and do not realise that they are gradually getting dehydrated. Drink at least six to seven glasses of water daily. Drink more in hot weather if you sweat a lot due to exercise and physical activity.

Pancreas:

The pancreas has several functions to perform in the body. Its primary role is to make hormones and digestive enzymes to keep blood sugar levels normal. The pancreas consists of a cluster of cells called islets which produce hormones that manage sugar levels. The two main hormones that are produced by the pancreas are glucagon and insulin.

Glucagon increases blood sugar levels by stimulating the liver to release stored glucose into the bloodstream when blood sugar levels are low. This happens during fasting or when one is unable to eat for different reasons, resulting in a very low-calorie intake.

The other hormone, insulin, does the exact opposite. Its function is to lower blood sugar levels by boosting the uptake of glucose from the blood into cells where it gets stored for later use for energy. Insulin also regulates protein metabolism, fat, and carbohydrates.

To keep the pancreas healthy and functionally optimal, schedule regular medical check-ups with your healthcare provider. Monitor diabetes or high blood pressure with blood tests, sugar level tests, and any other screening tests to evaluate your pancreatic functions.

Limit your intake of refined sugar, processed foods, and unhealthy fats because they lead to pancreatic stress.

To remain in top health, maintain the correct weight, exercise regularly, follow a healthy diet, avoid smoking, and limit alcohol consumption.

Keeping your three Musketeers—liver, kidneys, pancreas—in good health should be the top priority.

CHAPTER
13

HEART OF GOLD – THE TICKER

We live in an era where political heads of state have their own aircraft and are rarely if ever, seen on commercial flights. If I were working for an airline now, I would never get the chance to be a crew member on a flight that the Prime Minister takes.

Back in 1971, I was scheduled on a VVIP flight with Prime Minister Indira Gandhi on her flight to Moscow. There was always a frisson of excitement when we were assigned to a VVIP flight, but this was exceptionally prestigious. The flight was to depart from Bombay at 5:30 am for Delhi and then Tashkent and proceed to Moscow.

I was fully dressed in my uniform for my early morning pick-up when my father complained of a shooting pain in his chest that radiated up his left arm. This was not my father's first heart attack, so I was familiar with the drill. I placed two sorbitrate SOS pills under his tongue and gave him two aspirins and some water. He felt a bit better and got some relief from the pain. We had bought some time with the emergency medication, but I knew I had to rush my dad to the nearest ICU hospital.

It was 3:15 am in the morning. Fortunately, a taxi came to the next building to drop someone off from the airport. I got my father into the taxi and told the driver to take us to Petit

Parsi General Hospital in South Bombay on Warden Road. At that time in the morning, there was no traffic and soon, my father was admitted to the ICU under Dr Farokh E. Udvadia.

These were the days before mobile phones. In fact, I did not even own a regular phone—what we call a landline these days. I used the phone in the hospital to call Air India Crew Movement Control (Air India, Flight Operations office). I explained my emergency and my inability to join my crew members on the VVIP flight.

Much later, I came to know that my wife, Maloo, had already informed the driver who had come to pick me up that I had to rush my father to the hospital and would not be able to make the flight. The driver was very enterprising and took the initiative to do some scheduling on his own. He rang the doorbell of our Deputy Chief flight purser, Mr Peter Ryan, in the next building in our Air India staff colony and explained the situation to him. Mr Ryan jumped to my rescue by getting dressed, packed, and reported for the flight in my place.

The VVIP flight leaving Mumbai was delayed by fewer than 20 minutes. The Prime Minister, Mrs Indira Gandhi, and her envoy boarded the flight in New Delhi, and everything went according to plan.

I was very grateful to my friend and my boss, Mr Peter Ryan, who saved the day for me.

The next day, I received an urgent message from the Air India Admin Section to see the chief flight purser and explain the reason for missing an all-important VVIP flight. They set up a committee panel for this purpose.

I submitted a copy of my father's ICU admission form to the committee. The time of the hospital admission and scheduled departure of the flight were at the same time.

The inquiry panel was concerned and understanding of my father's condition I was let off with a mild warning for pulling out at the last minute from a VVIP flight.

A few days later, my father was discharged from the hospital, and we brought him home. The next morning, he was at the Elphinstone Parsi Gymkhana playing rummy with his friends in the club.

Later, I was told by Dr Farokh E. Udvadia that I had saved my dad's life by rushing him to the ICU in time. Any further delay would have been fatal. He also told me that in his years of practice as a cardiologist, my father was his only patient who had survived not fewer than five major heart attacks.

The heart is the most threatening perpetrator among all other major health issues.

When I was six years old, both my grandfathers died of a sudden heart attack within a short span of time. Another uncle died of a heart attack at the young age of 48. Most of my aunts and uncles from both sides of the family fell victim to major heart conditions. Just as certain names and characteristics run in families, a predisposition for early cardiovascular affliction seemed to run in mine. It appeared to me very early in life that I already knew how I was likely to die. I was fated to die from heart disease.

Compared to them, my father was lucky. He survived four heart attacks but succumbed to the fifth and passed away at the age of 64. I was 29 years old at the time of his death. I too suffered two massive heart attacks back-to-back in a matter of two days, followed by a triple bypass when I was only 52 years old.

As I write this book, I am 85 years old; 31 long years have passed since my open-heart surgery. I must have done something right in the last 31 years to still be here living my life.

I do not smoke. I rarely have a drink. I love food but eat small portions. When my stomach feels 75% full, I get up from the table. I have been following a diet plan known as "intermittent fasting" for the last 10 years. (Refer to chapter 23 on intermittent fasting)

My weight is constant. My lipid profile and my cholesterol levels are excellent. My lungs, liver, kidneys, and pancreas are absolutely well-behaved. My prostate is not enlarged. I may or may not wake up even once in the night to pass urine. Very recently, my blood pressure tended to rise a bit and stayed on the higher side. But with medication, it is under control.

I am in fine fettle. Age is a mere number.

A healthy heart is crucial for longevity.

Here are some indispensable steps you should take to keep your heart robust and in good shape:

Engage in physical activities and exercise regularly, at least five days a week. Take up activities that promote cardiovascular strength and endurance, such as brisk walking, running, swimming, or even dancing.

Adhere to a cardiologically sound and cardiovascular-friendly diet. Stick to a minimal or salt-free diet rich in vegetables, fruits, lean proteins such as fish and chicken, healthy fats, and grains. Partake in foods that are rich in nutrients, minerals, and vitamins that are good for your heart.

Maintain a steady weight as per the weight specified in charts according to your height and sex, the correct waistline, a good BMI (body mass index), blood pressure close to 130/80, and a pulse rate around 72.

Strive to be as stress-free as possible. Everyone has a certain amount of stress, but try to manage it as best you can. Practice yoga, meditation, and conscious and correct deep breathing techniques.

Associate with whatever brings you happiness and good cheer. "Mind your mind and you will be fine."

Go through your annual or biannual health check-ups. Know your lipid levels, blood sugar, and blood pressure readings. Do all your required blood work and monitor your heart health. Consult and clear any doubts about your present state of health with your healthcare provider.

If you are a smoker, give it up now. Giving up this self-demolition habit is not as difficult as it seems. All one needs is motivation and strong willpower. Stay away from second-hand smoke. Cigarettes are the biggest killers and the cause of heart attacks, stroke, cancer, and lung and mouth infections.

Drink alcohol in moderation. One or two drinks are as far as you should go. No more!

Limit your food intake to the minimum. Preferably avoid processed food, saturated fats, trans fats, added sugar, and a high amount of salt in your daily diet. Stay away from high-cholesterol foods that increase the risk of developing heart disease, even at a young age.

There are four life-saving medicines that could stave off a heart attack. They need to be mixed, crushed, and kept in tiny single cylindrical airtight pill boxes (or any small, single portable airtight pill boxes). I emphasise "boxes" in the plural because you should keep one in your pocket, and many others in alternatively and favourably in easy available places in the home. One never knows when, where, and who could get a stroke or heart attack. These small cylinder-type steel boxes are available on Amazon. They come attached to a key chain.

Take these four tablets, crush them all together, and place the powder in all the separate pill boxes. Attach them to your home keys, office keys, car keys, or motorbike keys. Always carry one in your pocket or your handbag, so that in any emergency it can be taken immediately with water.

1. Aspirin (Ecosprin) 325mg

2. Clopidogrel (Plavix) 300mg

3. Statin (Rosuvastatin) 40 mg

4. Nitroglycerine (Sorbitrate) 10 mg

The above combination is a potential lifesaver in an impending disaster. What is an impending disaster? Severe heart-clinching pain in the chest radiating to your left shoulder and arm, accompanied by profuse sweating. Open the pillbox and drink the contents (powder) down your throat, without delay. Time is the most important factor in a heart attack or stroke. With those pills in your system, you can buy some time to call your family doctor or an ambulance.

Making small changes in our lifestyle can make a world of difference to our life, lifespan, and longevity. Although the odds may be against you and your genes may not favour you, you can still win the battle by putting into practice a few fundamentals in the right place at the right time and persevering in the right direction to be in good health. Longevity is not merely about adding years to your life. It is also about adding life to your years.

However, the heart is often associated as the centre of emotions, particularly love, and is deeply entrenched in historical, cultural, and poetic folklore.

Here are some reasons why the heart is often connected to emotions rather than the brain.

The heart has been the symbol of love and affection in various cultures. The heart has always been a source of deep feelings.

When people experience strong emotions like love, anger, sadness, or stress, they often feel sensations in the chest. This will include an increased heart rate with a thumping feeling in the chest.

Or a feeling of warmth and friendship which creates a strong association between the heart and emotional experiences. And that is why we have phrases like "broken heart," "heartfelt," a feeling of a "sinking heart," and "I have given my heart to you," reinforcing the thinking that the seat of emotions is in the heart.

Also, the romanticism of love has led to the heart being seen as a vessel of true feelings emanating from the heart rather than the brain.

In summary, while the brain plays a critical role in thinking and processing, the heart continues to be viewed as the symbol of deep emotional connections.

However, physically speaking, heart failure is when one is declared dead, and it is the end.

The heart is the most physically active muscle in the body, pumping around 2000 gallons of blood per day. The heart rate in an average human being is about 65 to 75 beats per minute.

Did you know that a human heart beats more than 2.5 billion times in an average lifespan?

CHAPTER
14

KEEP YOUR LUNGS HEALTHY

Pinch your nose forcibly and close your mouth for a few minutes. As the Parsis say jokingly: "You will become a photo frame."

The inherent function of our lungs is to take in oxygen from the air we breathe into the bloodstream and ferry it to all the cells throughout our body. At the same time, carbon dioxide, a waste product, is eliminated through the bloodstream into the lungs and exhaled from the body. The lungs are at the helm of the swap and switch of oxygen and carbon dioxide in our body.

The lungs play a significant role in respiration, i.e., the process of breathing. During inhalation, the diaphragm and the chest muscles contract, triggering the chest cavity to expand, and the air is drawn into the lungs. During exhalation, the diaphragm, the thoracic, and the pectoral muscles relax, and the air is expelled from the lungs.

Therefore, the primary function of the lungs is to facilitate the exchange of oxygen and carbon dioxide between the air and the bloodstream. When we inhale, the oxygen in the air enters the tiny air sacs in the lungs where it diffuses into the blood, while carbon dioxide, which is the waste product of metabolism, is exhaled.

In addition to this exchange, the blood pH filters out small blood clots and thus plays a role in our immune defences by trapping particles in the mucus.

The lungs contain immune defences that protect against contaminants, polluted particles, and afflictions. The mucus produced by the lungs removes harmful allergens and foreign toxins, while immune cells destroy the microscopic organisms and clear the remaining waste from the airways.

Poor lung power leads to COPD, which is a persistent and long-standing lung condition that manifests in the form of breathing difficulties and airflow constrictions. It is often caused by long-term exposure to contaminating agents such as air pollution, cigarette smoking, or due to work hazards. Traffic policemen who spend hours every day on polluted roads or those working in chemical factories and underground tunnels encounter these work hazards. Symptoms of COPD are an incessant and deep-rooted cough, shortness of breath, production of abundant mucus, chest stricture, and gasping for air. Long-term COPD is a progressive disease that can affect the quality of life and lead to several additional contraindications like bronchial ailments, heart problems, and respiratory failure.

Deep breathing exercises go a long way in improving lung function and increasing oxygen intake. They also promote serenity and calmness. Deep breathing helps maximise oxygen and carbon dioxide exchange in the lungs. It increases the oxygen levels in the bloodstream that reach all organs in the body. This improves psychological and cerebral function and also improves energy levels and a sense of well-being. Deep breathing lowers the heart rate and blood pressure, giving a feeling of calmness.

Regular deep breathing exercises can bolster respiratory muscles and reduce anxiety and stress levels. These exercises should be performed by sitting comfortably in meditation mode with eyes closed.

Begin by inhaling deeply from the nose with the mouth closed for a count of four. Expand your abdomen as you breathe in. This fills your lungs with air for four seconds.

Hold your breath for a count of seven (seven seconds).

Very slowly focus on releasing and exhaling the air through a small opening of the mouth for a count of eight (eight seconds).

This is known as the 4-7-8 relaxed breathing method. This simple exercise will make you feel relaxed. It induces sleep and reduces anxiety. It brings your blood pressure down gradually over time.

Repeat this exercise as often as possible. You will see a great change in your all-around health, even if you are suffering from COPD or other respiratory ailments. It will increase the capacity of your lungs and put you in a state of relaxation. Try it!

Finally, maintaining overall lung health is very essential for ensuring that the most vital functions operate effectively, contributing to a high quality of health with a healthy body.

CHAPTER 15

EXCESSIVE GAS AND HEARTBURN

If you suffer from excessive gas, reflux, and heartburn, it is important to consult your family physician for an accurate assessment, medication, and corrective healing. The doctor can identify the underlying cause of your symptoms and recommend appropriate interventions to enhance your digestive well-being.

Excessive gas, resulting in heartburn and reflux, has several causes.

1. **Food and drinks related:**

   Foods that have a high carbohydrate content include specific types of beans, onions, and vegetables like cabbage, cauliflower, and broccoli.

   Carbonated soft drinks, products with milk derivatives, and artificial sweeteners.

2. **Digestive disorders:**

   Conditions leading to digestive problems, IBS, gastroesophageal reflux disease (GERD), and lactose intolerance can cause excessive gas and bloating.

3. **Swallowing air:**

   Most of us do not know that we can swallow air while eating, drinking, and talking. We also swallow air while smoking or chewing gum. This can lead to gas formation in our digestive system.

4. **Bacterial growth:**

   Abnormalities in our digestive area can lead to bacterial growth in the small intestine and gut which leads to gas and acidity.

5. **Medications:**

   Laxatives, antibiotics, painkillers, and anti-inflammatory medicines create distension, bloating, and an overabundance of gas in the digestive system.

6. **Smoking:**

   Incapacitates the oesophageal valve, allowing stomach acidity to rise into the oesophagus and cause severe heartburn and acidity.

7. **Obesity:**

   Overload of abdominal fat leads to overweight and obesity. This magnifies the burden on the stomach, which then causes gas, a burning sensation, an upset stomach, and acid reflux.

8. **Hiatus Hernia:**

   This type of hernia is caused by the retention of acid and food materials since the stomach gets compressed by the opening of the diaphragm. Food matter backs up, regurgitates, and reverses flow into the oesophagus causing intense heartburn. If left untreated, there is long-term impairment to the oesophagus. Leaking stomach acid brings on scarring and stomach ulcers which can bring about cell changes in the oesophagus, and intensify serious health complications, including the risk of cancer.

The best treatment for hiatus hernia these days is done by keyhole laparoscopy surgery.

The correct treatment for these causes depends on what contributes to these symptoms. Here are some common remedies for excessive gas, reflux, acidity, and heartburn:

1. **Lifestyle changes:**

   Elevate the head of the bed or use additional pillows.

   Avoid lying down or bending over soon after eating.

   Quit smoking and avoid trigger foods and carbonated soft drinks that bring on acidity. Maintain a proper weight.

2. **Eat small but frequent meals:**

   It takes 15 to 20 minutes for your brain to react to whatever you eat.

   Avoid large meals. Eat until you feel 75% to 80% full. After 15 to 20 minutes, your system will automatically feel full.

   If you eat until you are 100% full, 20 minutes later you will realise you have overeaten, and you will start feeling bloated.

3. **Antacids:**

   Over-the-counter antacids like Digene, Tums, Alka-Seltzer, and Rolaids produce instant relief by reducing the acidity in the stomach. They also give respite from stomach aches and indigestion.

4. **Proton Pump Inhibitors (PPIs):**

   Prescription meds or over-the-counter PPIs like Omeprazole and/or Esomeprazole can eliminate GERD symptoms and lessen stomach acidity. Zantac and Pepcid can also provide long-lasting reduction from colic pain and heartburn, and decrease hyperacidity and flatulence.

However, always consult your doctor first for a longer-lasting cure. Most long-standing ailments always need a medical professional's advice.

Anyway, to end this chapter on a lighter note.

There will be times when we are caught passing gas in a public place.

Here are some humorous ways to excuse yourself for passing gas or farting in a public place.

1. "Oops, sorry, I just released my inner ghost!"

2. "That was my inner trumpet solo. Sorry."

3. Play the blame game, like Mr Bean; point to someone nearby and say, "I think that came from there."

4. "Well, that's one way to clear the room." And pinch your nose.

A little humour can always ease the awkwardness and make the situation lighter and more enjoyable.

CHAPTER 16

FAMILY, FRIENDS AND RELATIONS

Dada J. P. Vaswani once said that your children NEED YOU more than the gifts you shower on them.

However, I say your parents and your grandparents, when they get old, NEED YOU more than all the gifts in the world.

Treat your family relations and money with equal respect because both are hard to make and easy to lose. Family is like a sitcom you accidentally star in. Everyone has a role, often exaggerated for comedic effect. You have the over-the-top mom who thinks everyone needs to eat more and needs a second or third helping.

And your dad repeats the same dad jokes everyone is tired of listening to. And if you don't laugh, he gets upset and tells some more of the same jokes.

Siblings? They are the live studio audience, who steal your French fries while laughing at your misfortunes. And let's not forget that one uncle, who always shows up at most mealtimes. And wants to know what is for dessert.

Family gatherings are like Bigg Boss reality TV shows where chaos, arguments, and laughter dominate.

So, let's face it. Whether it is family or friends, life is one big uproarious mess. And we are all trying to find overindulgence in the chaos. And who is marrying next?

Family, friends, and relationships bring closeness, happiness, a listening ear, a sense of belonging, warmth, anger, and harmony. They augment our lives with laughter, companionship, shared time, and good cheer most of the time. Especially when they are not fighting.

They create a sense of togetherness and community and foster meaningful relationships. With them, we share nostalgic memories, gaiety, and common experiences. Close relationships, whether platonic, passionate, or amorous, provide emotional support, affection, and attachment.

Family members provide unconditional love, support, assurance, and acceptance. They offer a strong foundation of belonging and are there for us through thick and thin, standing by with unwavering help and support. Family bonds share a joint history, similar backgrounds, and a way of life. They provide us with a familiar structure and direction to better our lives and overcome difficulties.

Friends offer different perspectives, give relevant advice, and help us broaden our horizons. A wider vision gives us possibilities to grow, leads us to self-discovery, and we evolve as better individuals, developing a higher understanding and self-awareness.

Good relationships bring meaning to our lives. They deepen our attachments, enhance our experiences, and amplify our contentment and joy in our lives. They are built on mutual respect, shared goals, and teamwork in achieving like-minded objectives harmoniously.

There is a common saying that since God cannot be everywhere, he created mothers. While it is more a poetic expression than a literal truth, the saying reflects the crucial role of mothers in our world. The comparison to God shows the omnipresence of motherly love and the divine impact mothers have on their children. It shows the unconditional love that mothers shower on their children. Mothers are the primary caregivers and nurturers in families.

Lest we forget fathers; they too play a very significant role in shaping their children's lives. Infusing life's lessons, instilling values, and providing for them as they grow.

However, by the time a grown-up man realises his father was right, he has a son who thinks he is wrong. So the chain continues.

Fathers are known to spend their life savings on their daughters' marriage. This is more common and prominent in India. Fathers often take heavy loans in order to appease and gratify the avaricious and insatiable, greedy parents of the groom, providing cash, gold, car, and furniture when their daughter gets married. Though the dowry system has been eradicated by law, it is still very prevalent in many cultures and societies.

It is said that "A son is a son until he finds a wife. A daughter is a daughter for life," and also that "Two daughters are better than six sons."

As the father of two daughters, I believe this and say this often. But it may not be true for everyone, nor is it right to generalise. Who came up with two daughters vs six sons? There is also a misconception that only daughters care for their ageing parents. I don't agree.

Sons also play a very active role in taking care of their ageing parents. The level of support, love, and care provided by sons, daughters, and other family members can vary widely. Personal relationships, personal and financial circumstances, and cultural norms play a crucial role. There is one saying that hurts my mind and soul: One mother can look after 10 children. But 10 children cannot look after one aged mother. If this is true, it is no wonder there are so many old age homes flourishing all over the world.

On this topic, I am reminded of a Bollywood movie, Baghban, released about 20 years ago that has stayed in my mind and memory as if it were yesterday. It was a tear-jerker that chilled the heart! The film stars Amitabh Bachchan and Hema Malini in lead roles, along with Salman Khan, Mahima Choudhary, and others. It is a movie about children in their adulthood who split their parents to live apart in their old age.

The story revolves around an elderly couple who have sacrificed their entire life for their children and raised them with love and care. However, as the parents grow old and retire, they have no assets or savings, since they spent it all on raising their four sons.

The four sons are obnoxious and cringe-worthy as are their self-centred wives. They feel that looking after both aged parents in the same house is too much of a burden. So they decide to split the parents into different homes so that they can take care of them in turns. The couple faces total neglect and mistreatment from their grown-up, married children and feel betrayed and abandoned.

Baghban explores themes of family values, generational conflicts, and the need to respect and care for elders. It is a poignant reminder of the sacrifices parents make for their children, who turn out to be ungrateful and selfish.

Baghban is the only movie where I cried. Although this movie is very old, I would recommend it to all my readers to watch it with their families.

As I was writing this chapter, I decided to watch the movie on Netflix or Prime Video. But it was not showing on either. So we saw it on YouTube, filled with ads and breaks. It is a movie worth seeing again and again. Once again, it brought tears to my wife's eyes, even though we are not in that situation and are looked after with love and care by our two daughters and their families. God bless them all.

However, it is good to know what happens to us after our funeral. In just a few short hours, the crying will subside. And your near and dear ones will be busy making arrangements for those who come to pay their last respects and will try to soothe your pain. They will be arranging food and drinks for friends and relatives. Some of your friends will be busy discussing current affairs over coffee.

Others will be apologising to your family for not being able to make it due to an emergency. Your employer will begin searching for your replacement. And in a few days, your children will go back to school, college, or work because the bereavement leave has ended.

Within a month, your spouse may be watching a movie, a comedy play, or a TV show, laughing as if you were never there. You will be forgotten at an unbelievable rate.

If people will forget you so easily, then who are you living for? You live your life thinking about what others think of you. When in reality, most people don't care as much as you imagine.

So live your life to please your creator, because He is the one you are going to finally.

CHAPTER 17

ALWAYS BE HAPPY AND STAY HAPPY

"How to be happy?" is one of the most searched topics on Google. Everyone wants to be let in on the secret society of eternal happiness. Everyone wants the inside scoop. Most people think happiness is a commodity that can be acquired.

"If I had more money, I would be happy."

"If I had a Mercedes Benz, I would be happy."

"If I had that beachfront house, I would be happy."

Material things will only give you fleeting happiness, but not true happiness. Happiness is not about getting everything you want. It is about enjoying all you have. It is in your own hands.

Be grateful for all you have. The grass is not always greener on the other side. It may only seem greener.

There is an old Hindi song in the film *Pyaasa* by the late Guru Dutt:

♪♪ 𝄞 ♪ *Yeh mehlon, yeh takhton, yeh taajon ki duniya.*

Yeh insaan ke dushman samajon ki duniya

Yeh Daulat ke bhookhe rawajin ki duniya

Yeh duniya agar mil bhi jaaye to kya hai?

Yeh duniya agar mil bhi jaaye to kya hai? ♪♪♪ 🎵 ♪

This world of palaces, crowns, and riches.

This society of enemies of humanity.

This world is hungry for wealth.

Even if you conquer this world, but your heart is broken, it would mean nothing.

So true.

"Uneasy lies the head that wears the crown."

True happiness comes from the inside. From within you. From your heart. It starts and ends with you. Happiness begins with you when you are satisfied with what you have. Not from your wealth, not from your job, and definitely not from how many friends you have on Twitter and Facebook, or how many groups you belong to on WhatsApp.

It is that easy. Not complicated at all. It is God's gift to us. Our bodies have the ability to produce happy hormones that keep us always in a state of contentment and bliss. Happy hormones are chemicals produced by glands in our body. They travel through our bloodstream and act as messengers in our bodies. They help to enhance our mood and maintain an upbeat attitude. They minimise anxiety and depression.

The hormones are dopamine, oxytocin, serotonin, and endorphins—also known as DOSE × 4. These four feel-good, happy hormones reinforce our physical and emotional well-being with help from us, by engaging in a few simple activities as a consistent routine. You can magnify and boost the levels of these feel-good hormones with simple life-altering daily practices and policies. There are lots of ways to self-produce happy hormones.

1. Practice meditation and yoga and exercise regularly, especially aerobics, swimming, and cardiovascular.

2. Go for long walks at least five days a week. Create a daily routine. Expose yourself to a daily dose of sunlight and fresh air by walking in nature, taking in the flora and fauna.

3. Make sure you get adequate restful sleep.

4. Maintain a healthy and nutritious diet.

5. Jive to your kind of music and dance to the beat if you feel your feet tapping.

6. Develop hobbies that give you kicks and thrills.

7. Do what gives you contentment, joy, and gratification.

8. Nurture and cultivate close relationships.

9. Hug and kiss your loved ones, connect with them, and love them.

10. Adopt a pet, even if it is only a goldfish.

Fine-tune your plan according to your personal needs. If you need a fitness trainer, nutritionist, or mental health expert for any of the above recommendations, go for it. The earlier you reach out for help and guidance, the sooner you will be back on track.

True happiness is a deep and lasting sense of contentment with what you have when you live every moment with a feeling of gratitude, fulfilment, serenity, and inner peace. It comes from a sense of resolve and purpose in being alive. Be thankful and count your blessings for what you have.

True happiness is often described as the innermost and deep-rooted sense of nirvana, peace of mind, and tranquillity that exceeds fleeting moments of gaiety and exuberance. It is not the absence of discomfort or difficulties, but rather the ability to find peace and gratitude amidst life's ups and downs. True happiness stems from significant attachments with family, friends, or even animals, and the ability to enjoy the smallest of things in life. It is the bliss that comes from pursuing your passions, not material possessions.

There will be times when conditions take you down and place their foot on your neck. At such times, don't struggle. Get your thoughts together and plan the week in advance. Try your best to be positive and optimistic, and know that this is only a momentary glitch.

Here are some lifestyle choices that negate and greatly diminish the production of happy hormones. Please don't do them.

Don't follow a lifestyle of loneliness and isolation. Meet friends, neighbours, and relatives as often as possible.

Don't close your mind to positive social interactions.

Don't stay away from an active lifestyle; like going for regular walks, visiting a gym regularly, or working out with aerobic or cardio exercises.

Don't ruin the natural balance of home, work, leisure, physical activity, and pleasure.

There are no hormones that contribute to gloom and doom, a negative state of mind, or sadness. Very low levels of serotonin, dopamine, and endorphins in the system bring about depression, mood disorders, despair, and loss of interest in everyday life. Cortisol is a hormone that is released due to fright or chronic stress, in response to tragedies, grief, financial difficulties, and other adverse events. Elevated levels of cortisol bring on anxiety and the same feelings as low levels of serotonin, dopamine, oxytocin, and endorphin do. The body has to walk a tightrope. Walk and maintain a fine balance.

Participating in activities that give you happiness will release an abundance of the DOSE x 4 happy hormones. Keep smiling, and the world will smile back at you.

Life laughs at you when you are morose and dismal. Life smiles at you when you are merry and cheerful. But life bows down to you when you make others happy and joyous. Be thoughtful, compassionate, and kind. *The more you do for others, the happier you will be. The more you give to others, the wealthier you will be.* People will not remember the work and effort you put in. They will remember how good you made them feel.

While laughter is the best medicine, it is not your mission to make everyone happy. You are not a bottle of Tequila!

Besides, if you come across a man who smiles when things go wrong, it is a sure sign that he has thought of someone to place the blame on.

In life, do not seek to make your presence felt. Just make your absence felt.

Finally, don't teach your children just to be rich. Educate them to be happy. When they come of age, they will know the value of things and not the cost.

Life is short. Spend it with people who make you feel loved and make you laugh.

CHAPTER 18

EARLY MORNING COCKTAIL FOR BETTER HEALTH

The early morning cocktail has been passed down to me and my siblings from my mother, who in turn got it from her mother. We down this cocktail several times a week first thing in the morning on an empty stomach. The ingredients are mixed and crushed together to form a paste in a small bowl by adding a large spoon or two of honey to negate the taste. Take a spoonful of the paste and follow up with a glass of water.

In case you are diabetic, substitute regular honey with sugar-free honey or jamun honey. After 15 to 20 minutes, you can have your morning tea or coffee.

The ingredients and their benefits:

Garlic:

Slice two or three cloves of raw garlic very thinly and crush them. Set them out in the open for a few minutes before consuming them. Garlic has a very sharp and pungent smell and is overwhelmingly pungent. When mixed with honey, the taste is neutralised. (Chapter 34 of this book is devoted to the benefits of garlic.)

Turmeric Powder:

Add a pinch of turmeric powder. (Chapter 35 of this book is devoted to the benefits of turmeric.)

Cinnamon powder:

Add a pinch of cinnamon powder. (Chapter 48 of this book is devoted to the benefits of cinnamon.)

Cloves:

Crush two or three cloves. (Chapter 39 of this book is devoted to the benefits of cloves.)

Ginger root:

Peel and crush a small piece of the ginger root into a pulp.

Ginger has been used for thousands of years for various ailments, like arthritis, colds, high blood pressure, and nausea. It has anti-inflammatory and antioxidant properties. It helps digestion and reduces symptoms of nausea and heartburn. Ginger restores and revives the skin and slows down the ageing process. Ginger root treats and prevents arthritis, and supports the gut to prevent intestinal gas, ebullition, and gut impairment. The compound in the ginger root helps the brain and nervous system.

Honey:

Add a spoon or two of honey to the above mixture paste to neutralise the taste of the strong ingredients.

Consuming honey every morning has a very refreshing effect on the whole body. It flushes out harmful toxins and improves digestion. Honey is a source of essential nutrition and energy. It has antibacterial properties, is very soothing to the throat, and is effective in the case of a cough. It inhibits coughs and asthma. Honey reduces inflammation and accelerates healing, especially when applied externally to wounds. It also facilitates heart health.

All of the above create a powerful blend of health benefits and flavours that have been cherished for centuries in various cultures.

This combination is known for its immunity-boosting properties and antimicrobial, anti-inflammatory, and cardiovascular health benefits, making it a staple in both cooking and natural remedies.

It is also well known for its ability to reduce nausea, improve digestion, enhance skin health, relieve joint pains, and promote overall wellness and well-being.

This blend is a delightful way to embrace nature's goodness in your daily routine.

Taking these combined ingredients in a paste on an empty stomach keeps you in fine fettle for a long and healthy life.

CHAPTER 19

ALZHEIMER'S, DEMENTIA, AND PARKINSON'S DISEASE

Alzheimer's, Dementia, and Parkinson's disease are neurodegenerative ailments that have a serious and significant impact on locomotor performance and cerebral and reasoning function, and deplete the quality of your life.

1. **Alzheimer's disease:**

    Research on Alzheimer's disease is not yet conclusive. It appears to be genetic and involves lifestyle and environmental factors.

    The symptoms begin with subtle memory impairment, which slowly progresses to disorientation and confusion, followed by an inability to perform daily functions, significant changes in personality, language impediments, and incapacitated judgment.

    Currently, there is no cure for Alzheimer's disease and ailments. However, there is ongoing research to comprehend the causes and discover the compositions at play that bring about the onset of this disease. Research is ongoing to slow down the advancement of Alzheimer's and manage the symptoms.

2. **Dementia**

Dementia is a disease associated with a rapid decline in cognitive tasks severe enough to impede and hinder day-to-day functions of life.

Indications of dementia differ depending on the underlying cause, but the symptoms include memory loss, disorientation, inability to cope with self-care tasks, flawed judgment, language issues, and major changes in personality and moods. Many people with dementia eventually reduce or stop eating affecting their nutrient intake.

Treatment for dementia depends on early diagnosis and timely intervention, cognitive therapy, lifestyle modifications, and supportive help from caregivers.

While everyone loses some brain cells with age, people with dementia lose far greater nerve impulses. Eventually, dementia damages the brain and the areas of the brain that control the body.

3. **Parkinson's disease**

Parkinson's disease is a brain disorder and causes major problems with mental imbalance, psychological health, sleep, involuntary movement, compulsive tics, pain, and other issues. In its later stages, it leads to muscle contractions, constrictions, painful body and limb tremors, and difficulty in speaking, walking, and locomotion.

Patients with Parkinson's disease suffer from increased pain in their neck and back, magnified and amplified due to motor dysfunction. As the disease advances, the pain becomes recurrent and continual.

Excessive daytime sleepiness is observed during waking hours. The disease can be managed to a limited extent by medication. At this stage, the medications are wearing off.

The worst thing about the disease is that it attacks the brain cell chemistry, stopping the capability to produce the happy hormones—dopamine and serotonin. These chemical hormones determine the moods, happiness, energy, and motivation. Without them, the patient goes further into deep depression and melancholy.

In the final stages of the disease, the patient needs round-the-clock care and assistance since they are confined to the bed with stiffness and frozen limbs.

At the end stage, it becomes impossible to swallow, leading to dysphagia and resulting in undernourishment, dehydration, aspiration pneumonia, and eventually death.

The disease can only be managed. Although there are treatments and therapies that can slow the progression of the disease, as of today, it may not be cured completely.

CHAPTER 20

EDUCATING OUR CHILDREN ABOUT GOOD TOUCH AND BAD TOUCH

Today's world is full of child victimisers, lechers, dirtbags, and sexual perverts who take advantage of innocent young girls and boys physically. Unfortunately, in most cases, these occurrences happen involving close relatives and trusted family friends in the neighbourhood.

It is imperative and crucial for parents, grandparents, caregivers, and teachers to educate children about the concept of good touch and bad touch to help guard them against molestation, prevent them from being taken advantage of, and secure their physical safety from a tender age.

Children must be made to recognise the difference between good touch and bad touch. Childhood education informing and explaining to them about good touch and bad touch empowers them to recognise and safeguard themselves from prohibited conduct.

It is very important for a child to receive and express fondness in a comfortable, relaxed, and safe manner. Any physical contact with a known or unknown person that makes the child feel comfortable, cared for, and safe is a good touch.

Good touches are reassuring and non-threatening, and make the child feel secure and happy.

Any physical contact that makes the child feel nervous and uneasy, leading to confusion, discomfort, and/or apprehension is a bad touch. This includes any touch in the private parts of the child's body, such as fondling and caressing against the child's will. It also includes undesirable embraces, cuddles, and kisses. Bad touches make the child feel alarmed and intimidated.

It is very important to teach the child to trust their own emotions and speak their mind to whoever they trust the most: parents, grandparents, and/or their teachers. It is necessary to educate our children and grandchildren that their body belongs to them and they have every right to refuse any touch that makes them apprehensive, uneasy, embarrassed, or ill at ease, even if the person doing the touching is a family member. We should have an open conversation and reassure them that they will not get into any trouble for speaking up. It is our responsibility to create a safe and caring environment where children can freely express themselves and share their concerns.

Parents can take many steps to protect their children from sexual abuse of any kind.

1. Educate your children on perimeters: Illustrate to your children that no one has a right to touch your child's body without their permission. And that it is OK to say NO.

2. Keep tabs on your children: Know where they are and with who they are with.

3. Tutor your children the various body parts' names. So they can convey and interact with you if something seems wrong.

4. Get to know the adults in your child's life like babysitters, teachers, school staff, and coaches. And check their references.

5. Be accessible: Let children know they can come to them if they feel awkward and disturbed or have any questions to ask.

6. Initiate family rules: Set up ground rules about privacy. Such as making changing rooms bathrooms and shower rooms as private places.

7. Enlighten yourself, about what is good and relaxed for your children to wear. And learn to trust your instincts.

8. Be aware of online risks. Keep tabs on what your children are watching on their i-pads and computers making warnings of exposure simpler to evade and spot.

This will encourage our children to communicate about abuse early, paving the way for quick intervention and prompt help. This is not a one-time, non-recurring conversation but an ongoing discussion as the child grows up and their understanding widens.

Let your child know that no one, not even their uncles and close family friends, has a right to touch them and make them feel uncomfortable. That includes hugs, kisses, and even tickling. It is important for the child to know that their body is their own.

Unexplained injuries and body marks are not the only signs of abuse. Fear of a certain adult, depression, sudden changes in sleeping and eating patterns, poor hygiene, hostility, and secrecy are often signs of a child being neglected, physically, emotionally, or sexually.

All parents and grandparents must know that this can happen to any child/grandchild anywhere and anytime. Caution at all times should be a must.

When talking to a child about abuse, listen carefully. Assure the child that he or she is not responsible for what happened. And they did the right thing by telling an adult, parents, and grandparents.

And finally, child abuse is a very deeply troubling violation of trust and innocence with lasting effects on victims and society as a whole.

Punishments for guilty child abusers should be severe and appropriately reflect the gravity of their actions, including long-term prison sentences and mandatory rehabilitation programmes after their prison terms. Society must prioritise a safe environment for all children, ensuring that those who harm them face quick justice and that victims receive the support they need to heal.

By the way, know that physical and sexual abuse are not the only means of maltreatment, but also children who are neglected by their parents and/or other caregivers who deprive the children of much-needed food, clothing, and care.

Children can also be abused emotionally when they are rejected, isolated, berated continuously, and beaten for their mistakes.

There are many kinder and more considerate ways to discipline our children. "Unconditional love" is one of them.

CHAPTER
21

THE GOODNESS OF REGULAR EXERCISE AND AN ACTIVE LIFE

In this day and age, when digital diversions, desk-bound jobs, and sedentary lifestyles are the norm, the importance of regular exercise cannot be emphasised enough. All you need to do is engage in some physical activity that you enjoy and love doing. It could be swimming, taking long walks, running, dancing, cycling, weight training, or engaging in any sports that you like. But the secret is to be consistent.

Incorporating a daily exercise routine and/or physical activity has a plethora of benefits that improve physical well-being and mental health and contribute to overall well-being. Additionally, if you introduce activities like yoga or tai chi, it will further improve your mental and physical state for the better. It improves muscular and skeletal health by strengthening bones and muscles, decreasing the chances of fractures and osteoporosis in later years.

Regular exercise has countless health benefits. It increases cardiovascular health, strengthens the heart, lowers blood pressure, and enriches blood circulation. It minimises the risk of obesity-related diseases like hypertension, diabetes, lung diseases such as COPD, and certain cancers.

It stimulates the body's natural mood booster, also known as happy hormones like dopamine, endorphin, and oxytocin. These hormones lower stress and anxiety and boost self-esteem.

Regular physical activity magnifies cognitive function. Daily exercise supports brain health due to improved blood circulation and growth of new brain cells, enhancing and sharpening memory and concentration. It gives you much better sleep and creates an adequate sleep pattern of seven to eight hours of undisturbed, peaceful sleep. You will wake up totally refreshed and ready to take on a new day. This improves your social interactions, leaving behind loneliness and promoting your spiritual well-being.

Engaging in physical endeavours regularly leads to sustaining a healthy weight and building brawny muscles and sturdy bones. You burn calories, shed weight, and improve coordination and symmetry. Active people are happier and live much longer and healthier lives.

To summarise, exercise has a multitude of health benefits.

1. Exercise will improve your quality of life.

2. Exercise will make you feel better and more relaxed.

3. Exercise can improve your sleep pattern.

4. Exercise can improve your brain function.

5. Exercise can help you manage your weight and burn fat.

6. Regular exercise can lower your risk of heart attacks, stroke, lung diseases, type 2 diabetes, and certain cancers.

7. Exercise can strengthen your muscles, bones, and joints.

8. Exercise can make your body recover faster from hospitalisations, requiring fewer and shorter bed rests.

9. Exercise will lower your risk of falls, especially in older adults.

10. Exercise will increase your good cholesterol (HDL), decrease your bad cholesterol (LDL), and also decrease your triglycerides.

11. Exercise would normally increase your life span. Keeping you "Fit & Fine at 99 and beyond".

In conclusion, regular exercise is absolutely vital for maintaining good physical health, augmenting good mental health, and improving the quality of life. Incorporating a regular fitness routine not only strengthens the body but also fosters vitality and resilience, making the future better and longer lasting.

CHAPTER 22

ACUPUNCTURE FOR HEALING AND WELL-BEING

Acupuncture is an ancient 2000-year-old healing and remedial art, implanted and deep-rooted in traditional Chinese medicine. It is a skilful and masterful technique that requires very fine, thin needles pierced into very distinctive and precise points of the body. While its origin is deeply academic, there is scientific validation that helps clarify how acupuncture fosters healing and overall well-being.

How acupuncture works:

1. Administration of the autonomic nervous system, which controls inherent bodily functions, can reduce stress and anxiety, supporting overall well-being.

2. Acupuncture can increase blood flow to certain areas by distributing more oxygen while eliminating waste products, which would expedite recovery from injuries and greatly reduce conditions like stiffness and muscle pain.

3. Meridian theory: Traditional Chinese medicine says that the body has corridors called meridians through which essential energy, "qi," flows (pronounced as "Chee"). Stoppages of this energy are thought to cause

disorders and ailments. Acupuncture aims to revive the flow of qi, energising clear-cut points.

4. Pain gate theory: Acupuncture can also work through the "gate control theory". According to this theory, certain nerves are affected and obstruct pain signals from reaching the brain, effectively closing the gate on the sense of pain. Acupuncture is generally used to treat chronic pains such as arthritis, knee and joint pains, and migraines.

5. Neurotransmitter release: Acupuncture stimulates the nervous system. When needles are inserted, they trigger the release of neurotransmitters, serotonin, and endorphins which reduce pain and promote a feel-good sensation of well-being.

6. Acupuncture also helps to cure digestive gastrointestinal infections like IBS by controlling digestive functions and decreasing stress-related syndromes.

7. Overall wholeness and well-being: Many people use acupuncture as a thwarting measure for maintaining good health and balance, supporting overall physical and emotional healing and well-being.

While acupuncture may seem enigmatic and mystical, its healing effects can be explained through modern scientific understanding and a combination of time-honoured and old-fashioned concepts of influencing the body's inflammatory responses, the body's energy flow, and neurological pathways.

Acupuncture can offer a comprehensive approach to health that can complement other mainstream medical remedies without side effects. As with any new treatment, it is important to consult a healthcare specialist or a professional to determine the best approach for individual health requirements.

Acupuncture is used for various health issues. Although scientific evidence varies, many people report benefits from this therapy. Here are some health challenges that can be helped with acupuncture.

It is a well-known healing procedure that has a very long-established tradition that bridges and combines the space between long-standing wisdom and present-day science. Despite its ancient origin, acupuncture is widely acknowledged in modern medicine due to growing scientific testimony on its known cures. It is a very effective tool and a superb engine for healing and intricate well-being.

Several theories and doctrines specify how acupuncture works wonders from a scientific point of view. Acupuncture involves inserting tiny, thin needles into specific points in the body to heal and soothe pain and other disorders. The insertion of needles at specific points in the body stimulates sensory nerves which in turn send signals to the spinal cord and brain. It promotes and propels hormones and neurotransmitters such as dopamine, serotonin, and endorphins. These hormones elevate moods and bring about a state of happiness and tranquillity. They also reduce anxiety and stress. They regulate moods and amplify the sense of well-being.

Acupuncture in specific points increases and improves blood flow in the body, carrying oxygen to all organs and tissues in the body, thereby reducing inflammation and enabling tissue repair. It also balances the nervous system. It guards the immune system, making the body more resilient against any infections and illnesses that come our way.

Acupuncture also regulates the digestive system, helping to alleviate conditions like hyperacidity, IBS, diarrhoea, dysentery, and even constipation.

Conditions like COPD, allergies, asthma, breathing problems, sinusitis, and low oxygen intake can be managed by improving respiratory and lung function with acupuncture.

Acupuncture helps in pain management—acute and chronic lower back pain, neck, knee, hand, and joint pain.

What I have written here stems from the knowledge I have gained from my wife and me being regular clients for several years of the very beautiful Dr Jasmine Modi, Acupuncturist and gold medallist. She is the head doctor, proprietor, owner, and Director of Acushastra Pvt. Ltd. at S.V. Road, Opp. Shoppers stop, Andheri, Mumbai 400058.

I would recommend seeing her for most ailments without hesitation.

CHAPTER
23

INTERMITTENT FASTING

They say, "Have breakfast like a king, lunch like a commoner, and dinner like a pauper."

Most people in the world think skipping breakfast is a bad idea. Almost a cardinal sin.

Not really.

From time immemorial, there have been diet plans, new diet theories, innovative diet concepts, and diets that claim to beat all diets, and on and on. Believe it or not, there is one very unique, recent, contemporary, present-day diet plan that is not very well-known. Intermittent fasting is a new game-changer without the "yes-no-yes, start-stop-start" yo-yo effect.

Choose the time period most suitable and convenient to you, depending on your mood, your working hours, your hunger, your rest and sleep pattern, and your energy levels.

For example, fast from 10 pm tonight until 2 pm the next day. The practice of 8/16 intermittent fasting involves eight hours of eating and 16 hours of fasting.

In the 24-hour day, choose a fixed eight-hour window for five or six days a week, where we partake in a reasonably healthy diet, and for the other 16 hours, we only drink calorie-free beverages like unsweetened tea, black coffee, and water during the fasting period.

Or say, you have a hearty breakfast by 9 am and an early supper by 5 pm. And you fast from 5 pm until 9 am the next morning. That would be feasting for eight hours and fasting for 16 hours.

This may sound difficult initially, but it is not. Our body is unbelievably unique, and very soon, it adapts itself, and we get used to the new schedule. Trust me, it will not be a problem at all. Numerous studies have proven that it can have very powerful benefits for your heart, brain, and your whole body.

Intermittent fasting is not only a means to shed excess weight and reduce the waistline, but it is also about burning bad fat. The popularity of this method of fasting has become very popular among those looking to lose weight and get rid of extra fat.

Besides losing weight and strengthening the immune system, it detoxifies the skin (inner and outer), making the skin glow.

With intermittent fasting, you eat fewer calories. Your digestion improves. You will also see a marked improvement in your sugar levels if you are diabetic, due to reduced insulin resistance.

Intermittent fasting improves and repairs the cells and removes waste matter from them. It also improves sleep, mental health, and clarity. It reduces oxidative stress and has an anti-inflammatory effect.

Intermittent fasting (IF) has gained popularity for its potential health-giving properties.

Here are some key takeaways associated with this diet.

1. Weight loss and fat loss. Intermittent fasting curtails calorie intake. Resulting in weight loss.

2. Improves insulin susceptibility which can significantly minimise the odds of acquiring type 2 diabetics.

3. Intermittent fasting can lower several cardiovascular risk factors, such as cholesterol levels, blood pressure, and triglycerides.

4. Intermittent fasting aids the cellular repair process—a process where cells repair damaged elements reducing the chances of various potential diseases.

5. Intermittent fasting can give rise to augmenting growth hormone levels which is valuable to replace fat with muscle gain.

6. It can reduce the chances of falling prey to cancer and improve the effectiveness of chemotherapy.

Those who find the 8/16-hour system difficult to follow can opt for a 10/14-hour or even a 12/12 cycle in the beginning. This is easier to accomplish because the 12-hour window is comparatively quite small, and most hours in that window may be spent sleeping. However, it is still effective because even in the lesser hours fasting window, the body will turn its fat stores into energy, which will release ketones into the blood, and this too will help in weight reduction.

If you find the decrease in your body weight is slow with the 12/12-hour window, you can slowly graduate to the 10/14-hour system. People who fasted for 16 hours a day showed more fat loss while maintaining growth in muscle mass with minimal exercise.

However, if obesity is the major issue, you can gradually move into the 8/16-hour system until you reach your desired weight. Then, continue with the easy 12-12 system.

The intermittent diet is a "win-win" situation for all because you choose what suits you best, and it is in your own hands.

For myself, I adopted the 8/16-hour system and lost 15 kg. I came down from 90 kg to 75 kg in two months. This reduction put my wife and daughters into a panic. I had to go through multiple tests to rule out any root causes like cancer for the weight loss.

To date, I continue this pattern and have maintained my weight at 75 kg. I follow the intermittent diet for five days a week, from Monday to Friday. Sometimes I have a regular cup of tea a couple of times during the fasting hours. My body has become so used to this system that it has become a way of life for me. There are absolutely no hunger pangs, and I feel very good.

Intermittent fasting is safe for most people. However, it is not recommended for women during their pregnancy and those breastfeeding their infants. It is also not recommended for diabetics.

While intermittent fasting can offer various health benefits, it is important to approach it thoughtfully.

Individual experiences and dietary needs can vary, and therefore, it is necessary to consult your healthcare professional before starting intermittent fasting and dietary changes.

CHAPTER 24

PSORIASIS AND HOW TO KEEP IT IN CONTROL

Psoriasis is a lifelong autoimmune inflammatory skin disease. It is hereditary and runs in the family. Visible symptoms are patches of thick, red inflamed skin with whitish-silvery scales that burn, itch, and may also hurt. Psoriasis makes the skin very dry, bleed, and sometimes crack. It is usually seen on the knees, elbows, scalp, and over the knuckles on the hands. If left untreated, it can spread from one part of the body to another.

Symptoms of psoriasis differ from person to person. Some people with this disorder often suffer from anxiety and feel stigmatised in public. The malformed and scaly appearance of the skin makes them feel embarrassed, especially when people they know mistakenly believe that psoriasis is contagious. Fortunately, it is not contagious and cannot spread to other people.

Most people who have psoriasis suffer from plaque psoriasis. This kind of psoriasis is likely to spread if the person does not seek early treatment. Psoriasis does not spread to another person, and touching a psoriasis plaque will not spread to the other person either.

I too was a victim of this menacingly unsightly disease in very limited areas of my body. It would flare up mostly in two places: my elbows and my knees. I was very fortunate that my plaque psoriasis was kept under control and never spread to other places on my skin that were visible.

For 38+ years of my life, I worked in Air India as a flying crew member (inflight supervisor and senior manager). Thanks to the uniform, the psoriasis was always hidden beneath my long sleeves and trousers. Otherwise, passengers and other crew members would have shied away from me, thinking this abnormally unflattering skin disease would spread and infect them.

Today, my psoriasis is almost non-existent. However, it has left behind very slight discolouration of the skin around my elbows and knees. Those spots are hardly noticeable now. They don't form any flakes, no itch, no burns, nothing.

I would like to name and thank the two lady dermatologists who have cured me of this horrible condition. My dermatologists, Dr Mrs Pramila Kanchan Aswani from Kalina, Santacruz East, Mumbai, and Dr Malvika Kohli from Pedder Road, Mumbai, are, in my opinion, two of the very best dermatologists today. They are gorgeous and I always thought could be playing lead roles in Bollywood. Instead, they chose a profession that heals all skin ailments and helps hundreds and hundreds of people.

Thank you, dear Pramila and dear Malvika. God bless you both.

It may not be possible to permanently cure psoriasis, but it can be brought under control to go into long-term hibernation. My psoriasis has gone into long-term remission. All that remains is a distant memory of the few areas where I had those ugly spots.

Here is a brief description of the treatments that helped me to rid the ailment. I was advised by my dermatologists to start on the following treatments:

1. Apply Lacsoft C Gel (Clobetasol Propionate and Ammonium Lactate Gel) once or twice daily, or as per the doctor's instructions, after a bath or shower to the affected regions.

2. Tablet Aprezo 30 mg [Apremilast tablets I.P. 30 mg] to be taken twice daily after meals, or as per doctor's orders.

3. Take one Foliate tablet [Folic Acid I.P. 5 mg] once a day.

4. Methotrexate tablets 5 mg once a day.

5. Use a coal tar (black) soap only for bathing or showering. Let the lather of the soap stay on the skin for at least 45 to 60 seconds before washing it off.

6. Use a shampoo that contains coal tar. Let it soak into the scalp for 45 to 60 seconds. Soap and shampoo can be applied at the same time.

7. Before going to bed at night, apply Moyzan (a light liquid paraffin emollient) to the affected parts. It will soften and hydrate your dry skin, leaving it looking radiant and fresh the next morning.

Despite your battle with psoriasis, always remember you are deserving of love, acceptance, and happiness. Keep a positive mindset. With the right care and proper medication, your psoriasis can be controlled. So, better days are ahead.

You are not your skin condition. Your resilience, your strength, and your inner beauty will glow brighter than a patch or two of psoriasis.

Encouraging someone who is dealing with the very visible challenges of psoriasis requires empathy and understanding.

1. Understand their feelings. Validate their emotions to let them know that it is OK to feel upset.

2. Localise on management. Discuss the various treatment options and address strategies. Remind them that many people have managed, controlled, and minimised their psoriasis very effectively. Scientific research for new treatments is ongoing and making significant progress. It is certainly not the end of the road.

3. Foster self-care. Motivate them to engage in self-care activities to enhance their moods, such as hobbies, pursuits, gentle exercises, and relaxation and recreation techniques.

4. Point out their inner strengths. Remind them of their toughness of character and the solidity they possess. Reassure them and pinpoint the different aspects of their life where they feel competent and optimistic.

5. Focus on an optimistic mindset. Concentrate on a positive attitude and self-acceptance. Reassure them that they are not alone. Many, many people in the world have much worse ailments and much more dreadful and incurable skin diseases.

6. If their temperamental health affects their day-to-day life, you can suggest and provide coping strategies and support.

7. Embolden open dialogue. Create a secure place for them to convey their feelings. Sometimes just talking about their inner sentiments and experiences can be very therapeutic.

8. Just be there. Sometimes just being present and tendering companionship can deliver formidable support. Let them know they are not alone.

9. I often used to meet people who suffer from psoriasis at dermatology clinics. I would spend additional time in those clinics explaining to them that I too was a victim of psoriasis and showing them the clearing of my psoriasis patches on my elbows and knees and the progress I have made over the years. It was always a moral booster for the patients.

However, every individual case is different and needs individual medical intervention through a medical provider or a dermatologist who will offer professional guidance to keep it under control.

I am living proof to hearten, enliven, and pep up individuals living with plaque psoriasis, reminding them of their inherent strength and resilience. With continued treatment, they too will be free of psoriasis, like I am today.

CHAPTER 25

UNDERSTANDING PSYCHOSOMATIC DISEASES

Psychosomatic diseases are physical illnesses that are significantly magnified by psychological factors like anxiety, nervousness, despair, and stress. These conditions have a deep and elaborate association between the mind and body. Unlike purely psychological barriers, these diseases are linked directly to mental and emotional stress and demonstrate actual physical symptoms without any actual physical trigger.

Here are some common causes and approaches to avoid them.

1. **Stress & anxiety**: Long-standing tension can lead to physical symptoms, such as headaches, digestive disorders, and chronic agony.

2. **Psychological torment and trauma**: Past traumas can exhibit fervent, poignant, and physical depression. Mood disorders can lead to physical debility as the mind and the body are intimately attached.

3. **Integrated and problematic conflicts**: Internal conflicts of animosity, guilt, and anger can bring about actual physical disorders.

4. **Ethnic variance and social elements**: Social and cultural elements can influence how one reacts to pressure.

5. Lifestyle and behaviour factors: Inadequate sleep, poor diet, and absence of any form of exercise and activeness can impart psychosomatic symptoms.

Strategies to avoid psychosomatic ailments.

1. **Regular exercise and physical activeness**: Engage in regular physical activities which will help to diminish stress and anxiety and enhance overall well-being.

2. **Stress and pressure management practice**: Relaxation methods, like yoga, meditation, and deep breathing to alleviate stress levels.

3. **Sensitive and despondent awareness**: Develop heartfelt intelligence by realising feelings. If required, talking to someone can help process emotions.

4. **Mind and body routine practices**: Examine practices like Tai chi or other holistic strategies emphasising connections between mind and body.

5. **Social assistance**: Build a strong network of friends and families, who can support emotional comfort during troubled times.

6. **Restorative counselling**: Seeking support from a mental health professional can be the tool to cope with whatever is stressing you and also to overcome emotional issues and recent traumas.

7. **Putting learning and knowledge into practice**: Understanding the connection between physical and mental health can empower individuals to take proactive steps for their well-being.

8. **Limit substance use**: Reduce or eliminate alcohol, drugs, and unrestrained caffeine.

By adopting these strategies, individuals can reduce the risk of acquiring psychosomatic ailments and promote a healthier mind and body connection. Therefore, there is a need to emphasise a holistic approach to psychosomatic diseases.

There are a number of psychosomatic causes that bring on actual physical symptoms:

Hypertension: Emotional, long-drawn-out anxiety and stress can be contributors to rising blood pressure.

IBS: Anxiety and stress can provoke or worsen diarrhoea. One may experience extreme cramps, abdominal pains, and/or dysentery.

Skin conditions and disorders: Psychological stress and anxiety can lead to skin diseases, such as psoriasis, eczema, and pimples on the face. At other times, hives and urticaria can also erupt without warning.

Asthma: Anxiety and stress can often bring about respiratory and breathing difficulties and also an asthmatic attack.

Chronic pain: Pain is often exaggerated due to continuous emotional, worried, and stressed-out minds.

Psychosomatic disease necessitates complex interactions between the immune system, nervous system, and the brain. Psychological anguish and suffering can alter how the nervous system processes pain, fear, and other sensations, amplifying physical symptoms. Stress and negative emotions inhibit immunity and make the body more susceptible to inflammation and open to various infections. Chronic stress energises the body's hormones like adrenaline and cortisol, which can impact various bodily functions resulting in genuine symptoms.

Today, psychosomatic diseases are on the rise, mainly due to increased stress in modern times. Constant technological overload, continuous information onslaught, and persistent digital connectivity lead to mental fatigue, leading to impairment of physical health.

Long working hours and high job demands lead to job insecurity and chronic stress, which in turn manifest into actual physical symptoms. Another damaging factor is the absence of real friends, resulting in social isolation despite digital connections on social media.

Diagnosis and treatment require a holistic and comprehensive approach. More so because the pain, feelings, and symptoms are real, although the main inner cause may be different and unreal. The treatment would typically involve an amalgamation of different approaches.

The first step would be to deal with stress and anxiety management through yoga, meditation, and mindfulness.

The next step would be lifestyle changes with light exercises, a healthy diet, and adequate sleep to improve overall health, followed by appropriate medications to tackle the underlying psychological conditions, after which the symptoms can be treated.

Recognising and treating the condition with comprehensive management, holistically and medically, becomes increasingly important. With an all-round approach, we can improve both mental and physical well-being, clearing the way for realistic and healthier lives.

CHAPTER 26

NAVIGATING DIFFERENT MEDICAL PRACTICES

Here is an overview of the different healing processes from ancient times to modern days.

ALLOPATHY (conventional medicines)

Allopathy is based on modern scientifically approved processes after years and years of research. It focuses on treating symptoms and diseases primarily through medications, surgery, and other interventions. It uses modern medical technology to diagnose, prevent, and treat various diseases.

It is usually the most tried, tested, and trusted treatment universally.

Allopathic medicine, in today's world, is the mainstream medicine practised throughout the world. It is the system for healthcare believed to be the best, as it is based on scientific evidence, scientifically researched for long periods of time, and is regulated by a neutral party like the FDA.

Here are the many proven benefits of the allopathic system of medicine.

1. Allopathy medicines use the best and the latest technology to diagnose and treat illnesses and injuries.

2. Allopathic medicines use various medical specialities, which allows practitioners to develop expertise in specific areas of healthcare.

3. Allopathy medicines are based on scientific evidence and research and years of clinical trials to ensure the efficacy and safety of the treatment.

4. Allopathy has highly qualified professionals, doctors, surgeons, radiologists, and nurses who have many, many years of skill.

5. Allopathy excels in emergencies that need urgent acute care.

6. The allopathy system has personalised professionals who can provide advice which is based on individual healthcare and specified needs.

However, when needed, allopathic healthcare often includes other alternative forms of medicine to treat some diseases and their side effects.

HOMEOPATHY

This form of alternative medicine originated in Egypt and ancient Greece by a German physician named Samuel Hahnemann, who started to experiment more and more and formed the theory that "like cures like", also known as "the law of similar".

That is when a substance in large doses causes certain symptoms; whereas in smaller doses, it can cure similar symptoms.

Today, homeopathy is used all over the world. Homeopathic remedies aim to stimulate the body's own healing mechanism.

Homeopathy is essentially a natural healing process. It concentrates on treating the patient more than the disease. It provides remedies to assist the patient in regaining lost health by stimulating the natural healing forces of the body. Remedies are individualised, based on the patient's specific symptoms and overall health.

Homeopathy uses extremely minute diluted amounts of plants and minerals that can help the body repair itself by promoting healing. In other words, something that brings on symptoms in a healthy person can treat an illness with similar symptoms.

The basic principle of homeopathy is that the substance that triggers a certain disease or an illness can also be used to treat that disease or illness. However, scientific evidence is mixed. In some clinical trials, homeopathy was no better than a placebo. In other clinical studies, researchers believed that they saw benefits from homeopathy. Therefore, more studies may be required.

Preliminary evidence shows that homeopathy may be very useful in treating diarrhoea, asthma, ear infections, chronic fatigue, pain, respiratory tract infections, colds, flu, coughs, allergies, treating childhood problems, and improving the quality of life in many other more serious ailments. However, one should not treat a life-threatening illness with homeopathy alone. They say homeopathy is a slow process. I personally think you must inform your healthcare providers to keep in the know if you are also using other therapies.

However, homeopathic medicines are usually diluted and do not have any side effects, and are not known to interfere with other conventional therapies.

AYURVEDA

Ayurveda is an indigenous ancient medical science, more than 3000 years old, founded in India. The southern state of Kerala is at the heart of this science due to Kerala's natural beauty, vast backwaters, green landscapes, and dense tropical forests. Kerala has a wealth of medicinal plants and herbs that are easily available to make elixirs and extracts for the preparation of a vast number of medicines from God's creations.

It draws attention to a holistic approach to health. The basis of Ayurveda is the universal connection of life's forces together with the body's anatomy, compound, and nature. Ayurvedic treatment takes a very personalised strategy in treating the root cause of health issues.

It employs herbal remedies, dietary changes, lifestyle adjustments, meditation, and yoga as methods to prevent and heal. The use of Ayurveda has both positive and negative facets.

Ayurveda herbs may bolster and enhance your immune system and help with immunity-related concerns. Ayurvedic preparations may help manage illnesses like diabetes type 2 to a certain point but in combination with other ongoing allopathic treatments. It can help to improve digestion issues, alleviate energy, lower stress and anxiety, and rid asthma and eczema, maintain weight. Ayurveda can help to lower blood pressure and bad cholesterol. It can help to speed up the recovery process from illnesses and delay the ageing process. Ayurveda may also help protect against heart diseases, rheumatoid arthritis, and prostate problems.

Ayurveda, it is said, chooses to eradicate the affliction from its roots. The treatment is straightforward, inherent, and holistic. It is known not to have any side effects because the treatment is a byproduct of nature.

However, the negative part is that Ayurveda medicines are not approved by the FDA in the US because Ayurveda has very little scientific evidence and undergoes minimal clinical trials. They do not meet the same safety standards as mainstream medications.

Beyond that, they may also contain harmful heavy metals like mercury, arsenic, and lead, which would probably interact with other medications and supplements and work against them, as well as create metal toxicity. Ayurveda medicines may also have pregnancy, breastfeeding, and prenatal interactions on the fetus.

I suggest it is important to research qualified Ayurveda professionals, reputable manufacturers, and evidence-based products and ensure proper diagnoses and monitoring.

Remember, Ayurveda medication should not replace conventional medical treatment without consulting a qualified healthcare professional.

NATUROPATHY

Naturopathy combines various natural therapies, including herbal medication, acupressure, acupuncture, and counselling. It emphasises the body's inborn ability to heal itself through natural therapies and lifestyle modification.

Naturopathy is a holistic approach to healthcare that emphasises the body's natural and inherent ability to heal and recuperate itself.

Naturopathic practitioners focus on the fundamental causes of health problems rather than just treating and alleviating the symptoms. This approach often includes a variety of disciplines, such as the intake of good nutrients, homeopathy, herbal medicines, physical activities, and lifestyle changes through guidance and mentoring, addressing physical, emotional, and mental health as well as lifestyle. Naturopathy aims to balance the harmony within the body.

Healing with naturopathy entails personal intervention plans tailored to the individual's unique health profile. Once the individual considerations are realised, they discuss with their patients to implement natural remedies that support the body's self-healing process. This would normally include stress reduction skills and a dietary regime to enhance nutrition intake to heighten and consolidate the immune system. It combines traditional healing practices with modern scientific tools, tests, and knowledge to foster overall wellness.

Finally, naturopathy motivates people to take an active role in endorsing and boosting life's long-term wellness of one's health through natural means as far as possible.

HEALING BY PRAYERS

Prayer is a spiritual practice that involves communicating with a higher power, a deity, a divine being, we all call God, the Almighty. Bhagwan, Khuda, Allah, our Lord, heavenly father, and creator of the universe.

Prayers take various forms, including spoken or silent words, rituals, meditation, and/or inner speculation, or even just plain good thoughts, good words, and good deeds.

Prayers are an integral part of religious and spiritual practices across various faiths and cultures. The act of praying from the heart involves communing with a higher power and seeking comfort, guidance, and intervention in times of need.

People pray for a multitude of reasons, such as expressing gratitude, seeking guidance and help, or finding comfort in troubled times.

They say, "Faith can move mountains." But I say, "Faith can move the world."

Faith in prayers is a very powerful force, offering hope when all else fails. This faith has a deep belief in a higher being to intervene in our lives, particularly in times of distress when all else seems lost. Faith provides a profound sense of hope, resilience, and comfort, which is crucial to the process of healing. Faith in the Almighty leads to a belief that He will heal and cure by His divine intervention. Individuals who have strong faith and belief and pray regularly often have better emotional and physical health outcomes.

When we are deep in prayer, we realise that we are not alone. Many people believe that sincere prayers can result in divine intervention, leading to emotional, spiritual, and physical healing. At such times, we realise there is a power at work beyond our understanding, beyond any explanation.

Believe in miracles because miracles do happen. Miracles are extraordinary events that go beyond science, beyond any medical explanation, and are often attributed to divine intervention. Accounts of miraculous healing have been documented throughout history.

There is a very common dialogue delivered by a doctor in many Bollywood movies: *"Abhi dawa ki zaroorat nahi hai, ab dua ki zaroorat hai* (Medicines cannot help now. It is time for prayers to the Almighty for His blessings)."

Then the doctor leaves the scene.

Next, after scenes of fervent prayers in Hindu temples, churches, fire temples (Zoroastrian agiaries), gurudwaras, and mosques, the sick are suddenly cured. The blind can see. The lame can walk.

The power of prayer is viewed as a profound practice that can bring hope, comfort, and a sense of connection to something far greater than oneself. We believe that prayer fosters a sense of peace, and emotional resilience, helping us to cope with anxiety and stress.

It is also a means of gratitude, thanksgiving, and seeking guidance. Research has shown that prayers can have physiological as well as psychological benefits, bettering mental and physical health and well-being. The sense of praying as a community, especially in groups, reinforces social bonds and support.

Finally, the power of prayers lies in its ability to strengthen faith and positivity to cultivate a much deeper conviction and trust in spirituality and the Lord above. The power of faith and healing transcends scientific understanding.

QUACKS

Quacks are fake individuals who pretend to be qualified medical professionals and carry fake medical certificates. These quacks set up medical health clinics, displaying false certificates and hoodwinking the innocent public. They pose a significant threat to the public by providing ineffective and sometimes dangerous medical treatment. Their misdiagnosis leads to incorrect treatment and harmful medications that worsen the condition and sometimes lead to death.

Fake doctors or quackery often prosper and continue their illegal practices and fraudulent businesses due to various factors.

1. Low-cost treatment: Quack treatment may be cheaper than conventional care.

2. Desperation: People seek quick fixes or cures for chronic conditions.

3. Lack of awareness: Patients may not verify their credentials and qualifications.

4. Quacks recruit a local army of cheats, con artists, and phonies who work to influence simple people through word of mouth.

5. Trust and credibility: Quacks use persuasive marketing and spread fake credentials. They are good storytellers. They exploit patients' emotions, offering hope. Their best trait is their tongue.

6. Social media: Quacks spread misinformation and attract victims.

7. They need to have charismatic personalities to flourish in their business. They are manipulative, exploitative, very deceptive, and scheming in their trade.

8. Often these fake, so-called quack doctors prosper because of the placebo effect. People are given sugar pills or just plain saline drips or saline injections, without any medication, but told they contain a medical and a magical potent that will quickly heal. The brain is fed on positive information that this medicine will make them alright in just one or two days (which in reality is actually nothing but a placebo). This belief makes the mind feel you are cured. The mind is so powerful that if you believe you are OK, you will feel OK, even for a short period of time. It is called the "belief system".

The mind is so strong. It can make you or it can break you. You can become mentally strong. Or strong mentally. You can have a hopeless end. Or an endless hope.

The placebo effect highlights the power of the mind in influencing health outcomes. It underscores the importance of beliefs, expectations, and the therapeutic context in the overall treatment process.

Some communities, especially in the villages of India, have a long-standing trust in traditional (folk) faith healers, often called "Vaidhjee". They are local practitioners, practicing their illegal trade.

Quacks exploit the ignorance and trust of the people, often charging lower fees than most qualified doctors to attract the desperate public to them, providing ineffective or dangerous treatments.

Remember, while laughter is the best medicine, it's always good to see a real doctor when you need to see one.

To summarise, I would say, stay well-informed, be vigilant, and prioritise evidence-based healthcare.

CHAPTER
27

CoQ10 – THE BEST HERBAL SUPPLEMENT

Imagine a range of mountains flourishing and booming with a billion medicinal plants, a zillion rejuvenating herbal products, abounding with a million beneficial supplements, limitless healing spices, numberless health-giving seeds, infinite restorative weeds, and a never-ending panacea of roots. Nature has provided mankind with all these amazingly magical resources spread across the globe.

I would place the supplement called Coenzyme Q10 at the apex of these mountain ranges. It is the mother of all supplements.

Coenzyme Q10 is a compound that is produced by the body. But as we age, our body produces less and less of it. CoQ10 plays several key roles in our body. Its primary function is to generate energy in cells in the body. Each and every cell in the body needs CoQ10. Luckily, we can also get it in supplement form. CoQ10 is recommended at any age to supplement a healthy diet. The capsules come in 100, 200, 300, 400, and 600 mg. Taken in adequate dosage (200 to 300 mg) is the most precious gift you can give to every cell in your heart, in your brain, and to your whole body.

Taking a CoQ10 supplement daily offers unimaginable health benefits.

1. Heart health: CoQ10 is known to support cardiovascular health by improving blood vessel functions and lowering blood pressure.

2. Energy production: CoQ10 plays a very crucial role in the production of energy cells in your whole body, which enhances overall energy levels.

3. Cognitive function: There is undisputed evidence that CoQ10 supports brain health and improves cerebral and psychogenic function. It also supports neuroprotection.

4. Antioxidant protection: It acts as a powerful antioxidant, helping to neutralise free radicals and reduce oxidative stress, which protects cell damage and reduces inflammation.

5. Improves exercise performance: CoQ10 enhances stamina, endurance, and physical performance making it very beneficial for athletes and active individuals.

6. Supports muscle health and reduces muscle cramps.

7. Supports skin health and reduces signs of ageing.

8. Helps manage migraines and chronic fatigue syndrome.

9. Supports eye health and reduces the risk of age-related macular(AMD) degeneration. AMD affects the centre of the retina which causes blurry and fuzzy vision and may also cause blindness.

10. May improve fertility and reproduction.

11. May slow Parkinson's and Alzheimer's disease progression.

12. May improve insulin sensitivity and sugar levels.

13. May support treatment for certain cancers, (eg. prostate, breast, and lung).

CoQ10 alleviates symptoms of congestive heart disease. Research also suggests that when taken with some other nutrients like Omega 3 fish oil, raw garlic, and olive oil, it greatly helps recovery in people who have had previous heart attacks, open-heart surgeries, bypasses, and/or corrective heart valve surgeries. It also maintains normal blood circulation and a good heart rhythm.

CoQ10 helps maintain normal levels of triglycerides and improves the good cholesterol HDL levels. CoQ10 is also known to counteract the adverse effects of statins (cholesterol medications).

CoQ10 helps normal brain function and improves the immune system. It improves fertility in men and women.

CoQ10 is directly linked to anti-ageing properties. It is definitely the best supplement for improving heart health and longevity.

My daughter Jennifer's three pet dogs, Muffin, Crystal, and Jacky, were brought to India from Texas. She fed them with regular dosages of CoQ10 in their diets. Their energy and fitness levels stayed at an optimum level, and they outlived by far the normal lifespans for their Bichon Frise breed.

I absolutely, strongly, and wholeheartedly recommend this supplement to all my readers and their families. CoQ10 is a supplement highest on my list to augment, rejuvenate, and a shot in the arm for longevity. There is no better supplement to breathe a brand new life into you.

Buy it from Amazon or wherever today!

If a man gives you a fish, you will eat fish for one day.

If he teaches you how to fish, you will eat fish every day.

CHAPTER 28

OMEGA FISH OIL SUPPLEMENTS

Let your food be thy medicine and not medicine thy food. Seafood is one of the best things to consume on a regular basis. You will live a very long life in good health.

Eskimos and Japanese have very long lifespans, mainly because their staple diet has always been fatty oily fish. If you do not eat a lot of oily fish like salmon, sardines, anchovy, tuna, and herrings, you must augment your meals with fatty acid supplements on a daily basis.

If CoQ10 is the mother of all health supplements, Omega 3 fatty acids capsules would be the father of all supplements. These capsules are exceedingly helpful to enrich, support, and improve the health of your entire body.

Fish oil is an excellent source of Omega-3 fatty acids and the most commonly used dietary supplement. There is nothing better for your heart, brain, and body than Omega-3 fatty fish oil capsules.

Omega-3 oil helps to prevent plaque formation and hardening of the arteries. Thereby, it lowers your blood pressure. It increases your good cholesterol (HDL) and lowers your bad cholesterol (LDL). It also decreases your triglycerides by 25% to 30%. Omega-3 goes a long way in improving your liver function.

Fish oil supplement is a Polyunsaturated Fatty Acid, commonly known as PUFA. The body cannot make the PUFA nutrient for itself. This nutrient benefits people with many different skin conditions and skin ailments, like dry skin, scaly skin, itchy skin, psoriasis, acne, and dermatitis.

Fish oil supplements inhibit inflammation and more. Omega-3 reduces inflammation in the body and promotes anti-ageing.

Fish oils contain vitamins A and D and selenium. Vitamin A contains an antioxidant, retinol, which softens the skin, hydrates the cells in the skin, and promotes total skin healing. The skin is the largest organ in the human body.

Research has shown that good fish oils contain 180 EPA (Eicosapentaenoic) and 120 DHA (Docosahexaenoic), which are long-chain Omega polyunsaturated fatty acids, known as Omega-3s. Our body very much needs EPA and DHA in Omega-3 to function properly in every stage of our lives. It is advisable for pregnant ladies, lactating and breastfeeding mothers to consume DHA in particular from Omega fish oil throughout the pregnancy and during the breastfeeding of their infants.

Consumption of Omega-3 supports overall wellness, including the brain, heart, skin, eyes, and much more. It is a very important nutrient and is a must to incorporate it into our daily diet or as a daily supplement.

Taking Omega fish oil supplements daily can offer several incredible and unimaginable benefits, primarily due to the essential fatty acids they contain.

Here is a breakdown of the goodness of Omega-3 fish oil supplements.

1. Heart health: Omega-3 fatty acids are famously known to support cardiovascular health like no other supplements.

It can greatly reduce the formation of triglycerides and bad cholesterol (LDL) in the blood.

2. Decreases plaque formation: Regular intake can lower blood pressure by reducing plaque formation in the blood vessels contributing to unrestricted blood flow.

3. Powerful anti-inflammatory properties: They help to reduce rheumatoid arthritis and painful chronic inflammation conditions, which are linked to various heart diseases, cancer, and autoimmune disorders.

4. Skin health: Omega-3 can help to retain moisture due to hydration. Reduce acne and other skin conditions.

5. Brain health: Omega-3 fatty acids are essential to reduce the risk of getting Alzheimer's and Dementia and also for maintaining cognitive function.

6. Eye health and vision maintenance: Omega-3 can help to protect against age-related macular degeneration (AMD) and other eye disorders.

7. Support for pregnancy and newborn: Adequate Omega-3 fatty acids are crucial for the brain and eye development of the foetus. Omega-3 capsules may also help to prevent postpartum depression in new mothers. Considering the goodness of our health, Omega-3 is priceless and should be a part of our daily herbal intake. I again beseech my readers and their loved ones to start taking them asap.

My aim and my ambition in writing this book are not just to share knowledge. It is to arouse and instil action, revolutionise lives, and make a fitter and healthier world for everyone.

CHAPTER 29

VITAMIN K2

Vitamin K2, one of the most underrated vitamins, is known as the clotting vitamin.

Without vitamin K2, clotting would not be possible, and with any injury, we would bleed to death. It helps our body produce various proteins to aid blood clotting. If one is on Warfarin, Aspirin, Plavix, or any other blood thinner, a cut or an open wound can result in internal or external bleeding. Vitamin K2 helps the blood to clot and reverses the blood-thinning process.

Vitamin K is less known than many other vitamins, like A, B, C, D, and E, for several reasons.

1. Less publicity: Other vitamins are commonly mentioned in the framework of health and wellness due to the roles they play in the growth of the body, development, hormone control, nerve health, immunity function, bone health, blood clotting, energy creation, wound restoration, and helping cells and organs to do their jobs as needed.

2. Confusion of understanding: There are two forms of vitamin K (K1 and K2) and their different

functions contribute to a lack of understanding in the general public.

3. Adequate consumption through their food: Most people get their vitamin K through their diet without knowing it, which leads to a lack of debate about its significance compared to other vitamins that are frequently inadequate.

4. Recorded emphasis: The classification and the discovery of vitamins often advertised which have more immediate health effects. Vitamin K's blood clotting role may not have been so obvious initially.

However, while vitamin K2 is crucial for good health, it may have a lower profile when compared to other vitamins. This could be due to a combination of dietary, historical, and lack of awareness.

The intake of vitamin K2 daily reduces the chances of a heart attack by 60% since it blocks the progression of thickening and stiffening of the arterial walls. Vitamin K2 assists in building strong bones and teeth. People with low-density brittle bones are very prone to fractures, especially in old age. It also prevents the early onset of osteoporosis. Vitamin K2 is also an excellent nutrient for maintaining proper heart and brain function and skin health.

Vitamin K2, in combination with Vitamin D3, helps to lessen menstrual pains.

Vitamin K2 works miracles on the skin. It improves the skin's ability to heal itself—heal bruises and wounds quickly and effectively. Additionally, it helps the skin to slow down the ageing process and prevents premature ageing. Collagen and elastin prevent wrinkles. As a result, Vitamin K2 is used in the manufacture of many facial creams and lotions to apply under the eyes to lighten and brighten dark circles and boost the elasticity of the skin.

A very recent study has found that vitamin K2 acts as an antioxidant that could prevent the onset of Alzheimer's disease and improve mental ability.

Vitamin K2 is a must for the body to glow, grow, slow the ageing process, function normally, heal, and beautify the skin.

Vitamin K2 is found in many green vegetables, Brussels sprouts, broccoli, cabbage, spinach, kale, lettuce, cauliflower, tomatoes, sweet potatoes, and carrots. It is also found in many fruits like avocado, prunes, grapes, blueberries, and even apples, although to a smaller extent.

NB: Vitamin K should NOT be mistaken for Potassium.

CHAPTER
30

VITAMIN D3

Vitamin D3 is well known as the sunshine vitamin.

Vitamin D can be obtained from exposure to the sun, food fortification, or through supplements. However, too much vitamin D can cause toxicity. The tolerable upper level is 4,000 IU for adults.

People living close to the equator benefit from the God-given gift of plenty of sunshine, while populations close to the North Pole and the South Pole suffer from a paucity of sunlight. They need to supplement the loss by adding additional Vitamin D3 to their diet.

Cod liver oil has the highest content of vitamin D3. Fatty fish like salmon, sardines, herrings, and mackerel have a very high content of Vitamin D3, as do the yolk of eggs, broccoli, spinach, kale, papaya, and oranges. Fortified dairy products like cheese, milk, and yoghurt also have Vitamin D3.

It is strongly recommended to take Vitamin D3 supplements daily if one does not get it through exposure to sunlight or diet. It has numerous and incredible health benefits.

Vitamin D3 plays a key role in calcium assimilation, which is pivotal for preserving healthy, strong bones, teeth, and nails.

Adults and children who are low in the nutrient D3 have low calcium and phosphorus levels in their bones, which leads to an increased risk of bone fractures, joint weakness, and muscle pains. High calcium levels in the body prevent accidental splintering and cracking of weak bones. Low calcium content in the bones brings on a condition called Osteoporosis. Calcium deficiency leads to rickety and brittle bones, osteoporosis in adults, and rickets in children. Severe deficiency of calcium can cause osteomalacia, which can result in multiple and frequent bone fractures caused by the smallest of injuries and falls.

Older people fracture their hip bone after a fall and are bedridden. Bones take a very long time to heal in old age. The "25-Hydroxy vitamin D" test is the most reliable way to measure how much vitamin D is in the body. Bone density checks evaluate the amount of calcium in the bones. We don't want a fractured hip or a broken back, do we?

Calcium supports the formation of keratin, which is a building block for nails. Good calcium levels contribute to overall nail health, and a lack of it leads to weak, thin, and brittle nails.

Vitamin D3 is important for skin health, which incidentally is the largest organ of the body. The skin helps to keep the moisture inside to inhibit dehydration. It balances the creation and procreation of cells present in the epidermis, the external surface layer of the skin. These cells are essential for preserving and safeguarding the work of the skin barrier and also take in the sun's rays.

Taking vitamin D3 daily helps enhance the immune system and the cardiovascular system and regulates moods. It regulates blood pressure and reduces the risk of cardiovascular diseases. It also plays a role in weight regulation and management.

There is evidence to suggest that vitamin D3 safeguards the body from colon, prostate, and breast cancer. It reduces the advancement of cancer cells and diminishes cell growth.

Vitamin D deficiency can lead to several health problems.

1. Osteoporosis: A condition where bones become weak and fragile and may break easily.

2. Falls: A much higher risk of falls in old age.

3. Sarcopenia: A progressive loss of muscle mass and strength.

4. Cardiovascular disease: Cardiovascular disease has been linked to vitamin D deficiency.

5. Diabetes: Diabetes is also linked to vitamin D deficiency.

6. Depression: Vitamin D deficiency can also bring on a state of depression.

7. Cancer: Vitamin D deficiency has been linked to even cancer.

So, make sure you get your 3000 to 4000 IU of vitamin D daily.

After my first book was published, some friends asked my wife which book, among all the books she had read, was most helpful and liked by her.

Without skipping a beat, Maloo replied, "Noshir's cheque book!"

She is proof that the brain works really fast with regular intake of olive oil.

CHAPTER

31

EXTRA VIRGIN OLIVE OIL

More and more people now know about the perks of switching to olive oil. Extra virgin olive oil, a staple in Mediterranean cuisine, is renowned for its numerous health benefits and culinary versatility. Packed with anti-inflammatory properties and antioxidants, it supports overall wellness and may reduce the risk of chronic diseases. Being rich in monounsaturated fats, it promotes robust heart health by helping to reduce triglycerides and cholesterol levels. Its flavour enhances a variety of dishes, making it a popular choice for cooking, dressings, marinades, and salads.

It is a well-known fact that the Mediterranean diet is rich in extra virgin olive oil, antioxidants, fish, fruits, legumes, and vegetables, which brings on additional high-density lipoprotein i.e., the good cholesterol (HDL). As HDLs are guaranteed to perform much more effectively, extra virgin olive oil further helps to get rid of the excess bad cholesterol (LDL) from the blood in your arteries.

You can cook in olive oil. The greatest advantage of spending a little more money on extra virgin olive oil is that when you add it to salads or even have a small tablespoon of it directly, it will boost your heart health significantly.

Additionally, regular use of extra virgin olive oil most definitely gives better skin health and improves digestion, making it a very valuable addition to any kitchen.

Olive oil significantly improves the function of your blood vessels and inflammatory markers, which reduces the bad cholesterol (LDL) and thereby reduces the risk of getting heart disease.

Research has shown that extra virgin olive oil in your diet lowers your blood pressure and keeps your arteries from hardening, thereby safeguarding your heart. It helps maintain better blood flow and clears all the fat and refuse from the arteries.

Extra virgin olive oil may also bring about the death of cancer cells.

For personal appearance, it is the best-softening moisturiser. You can apply it to your face to bring on a glow and smooth the tone of your skin. You can massage your scalp with it and apply it to your hair for thicker hair growth. Olive oil and almond oil are now the preferred oils for a full-body massage.

I would recommend 100% natural Figaro cold-pressed extra virgin olive oil. This high-quality product is now available in India and made from the finest olives from Spain. Use it daily in cooking, as a homemade salad dressing, on parathas, or mixed with butter and poured liberally on hummus, and even gulp a small spoon or two every day. You will see your life change for the better.

Viva Espana!

CHAPTER

32

SEEDS

See the beauty of nature. A small seed grows into a magnificent and colossal tree.

Seeds are the embryo for a robust tree to grow and are filled with unlimited nutritional value. Brimming with healthy polyunsaturated fats, monounsaturated fats, and loads of fibre plus a plethora of important minerals, vitamins, and antioxidants.

Imagine the incredible advantages of adding seeds to your diet. They provide important nutrients and major health benefits. Seeds offer a quantum leap to better health and well-being.

Being high in good fat and protein, and replete with fibre, seeds are the ideal snack and fill you up faster. They also give you extra vigour and vitality. They are very good alternatives to snacks in between meals when you feel the pangs of hunger. Instead of reaching for high-calorie snacks and adding unhealthy calories, partaking in delicious and varied roasted seeds at snack time can be a far better choice. However, it is best to have them in small quantities and frequently if you so desire.

When combined with a balanced diet, seeds can effectively lower bad cholesterol levels, sugar in the blood, and blood pressure. Seed consumption is known to contain insoluble fibre, which assists in taking care of visceral health.

Seeds are stored and used throughout the year. The best thing about seeds is they can be used to raise crops as per the requirements of the season and the availability of the fields and manpower.

Chia, sunflower, and flax seeds are rich in Omega fatty acids, which improve good cholesterol and control inflammation, thereby enhancing the overall functioning of the heart.

Among the many distinctive seeds to consider for your nutritional stockpile are:

1. **Pumpkin Seeds:**

   Pumpkin seeds contain phosphorus and omega-6 fats, monounsaturated fats, and phytosterols that assist in lowering blood cholesterol.

2. **Flax Seeds:**

   A rich source of fibre and omega-3 fats, particularly alpha-linolenic acid (ALA). It is best to grind flax seeds to access the omega-3 within the shell.

3. **Chia Seeds:**

   Like flax seeds, chia seeds overflow with fibre and omega-3, accompanied by a host of other important nutrients.

   They are a treat in milkshakes, falooda, and desserts.

4. **Sesame Seeds: (black and white)**

   Sesame seeds help to reduce inflammation and mitigate oxidative stress, which is most important for various health conditions. They have been known for centuries to possess many additional benefits.

Sesame seeds are known to build healthy bones and they also help the digestion process.

5. **Sunflower Seeds:**

Rich in protein, vitamin E, and monounsaturated fats, sunflower seeds also help to reduce inflammation, thereby reducing the risk of heart disease.

6. **Hemp Seeds:**

They are loaded with increased vegetarian protein content. Hemp seeds provide a complete protein source with all essential amino acids.

7. **Alfalfa Seeds:**

For vegetarians, alfalfa seeds are a big boon due to their high protein content. They protect against cellular damage.

Alfalfa seeds are priceless when it comes to fulfilling daily nutrition. They are the best seeds for building immunity as they are a rich source of antioxidants.

8. **Watermelon Seeds:**

When you eat watermelon, don't throw away the seeds. Watermelon seeds are an excellent source of zinc, iron, and magnesium. Eating them roasted is a deliciously healthy snack.

The next time you think of a seed, remember it contains the embryo of a small plant or a towering tree.

If a Genie suddenly appeared and asked me to choose between our ancient Indian Kohinoor diamond, the largest cut diamond in the world that is now among the crown jewels in England, or a lifetime supply of Tru Niagin, can you guess which one I would choose?

CHAPTER

33

TRU NIAGEN FOR LONGEVITY – VITAMIN B-3

If CoQ10 is the mother of all herbs, and Omega-3 is the father of all supplements, Tru Niagin would be the God of all supplements and vitamins.

In the year 2004, Dr Charles Brenner discovered a very rare and unique form of vitamin B3, which is exceedingly uncommon to find in nature - Nicotinamide Riboside (NR) or Niagen. It is the vitamin that has been proven to aid the longevity of mankind. It has the ability to increase the levels of **Nicotinamide Adenine Dinucleotide** (NAD), which is a molecule that is extremely vital to sustain life as we know it. Its contribution to healthy ageing is phenomenal. It is truly the key to life.

Nicotinamide Riboside is marketed as Tru Niagen and is a supplement true to its name—the God of all supplements. It helps improve our cellular function, our metabolism, and overall well-being. The total nutritional support of this compound may even reverse the ageing process and promote lifespan like no other supplement to date. However, its full potential is still under research.

For optimum results, Tru Niagen needs to be taken in 300 mg capsules every morning at the same time if possible, with or without food. It is priced at about US$50+ for a month's supply of 30 capsules. Tru Niagen Vitamin B3 is additionally enhanced with vitamin D, vitamin C, zinc, and curcumin.

Tru Niagen is a dietary supplement designed to boost levels of Nicotinamide Adenine Dinucleotide (NAD+), a vital coenzyme that helps DNA repair, cellular function, and energy production. Its key ingredient is a form of vitamin B3 that increases the levels of NAD+.

By enhancing NAD+ availability, Tru Niagen ensures healthy ageing, supports cognitive health, and improves metabolic function on a different level. All users understand and value its potential to upgrade overall vitality and energy levels, making it a very popular choice to enhance one's wellness regime.

Tru Niagen is a Kohinoor diamond for your health and longevity. Intake of one 300mg capsule daily will do wonders for your health and your life.

Trust me. My wife and I, despite our age and our not-so-good health genes, are both 85 and kicking.

A clove or two of garlic a day keeps the Devil away.

CHAPTER 34

GARLIC

Did you know that onion and garlic are in the same subfamily called Allium?

Garlic is considered a vegetable and not a herb or a spice.

Garlic has innumerable health benefits. If everything about the little vegetable had to be listed, it would need a separate book.

Garlic has been a major part of cooking in Indian, Italian, Mediterranean, and Chinese cuisine for centuries. This vegetable has medicinal and curative properties because of its antibacterial, antimicrobial, and antiseptic nature.

Raw garlic can keep cough and cold infections away. Eating one or two crushed garlic cloves every morning on an empty stomach can work miracles on our system. It can prevent heart blockages. Garlic helps to reduce the stickiness in the platelets of the blood and thus prevents the clotting of blood which would ultimately reach the heart through the arteries and cause a heart attack or reach the brain and result in a stroke. Garlic also lowers blood pressure.

Allicin, a compound found in garlic that helps to reduce bad cholesterol (LDL), has potent antibacterial, antiviral, and antifungal properties, which can help strengthen the immune system. Raw garlic is celebrated for its impressive health benefits, making it a powerhouse in nutrition.

Another good thing about garlic is that it improves problems with the digestive system. It reduces inflammation in the stomach and intestines by protecting the good bacteria and destroying the bad bacteria.

Blood sugar levels come down in type 2 diabetics with the consumption of raw garlic in the morning. Garlic is also rich in antioxidants, which fight oxidative stress and in turn, reduce and counter acquiring chronic diseases.

Additionally, it has been linked to much-improved heart health by reducing bad cholesterol and triglycerides, clearing and cleaning the blood vessels, and lowering blood pressure. Its anti-inflammatory and antioxidant properties can support overall wellness.

Garlic also promotes brain health. It is known to prevent dementia and Alzheimer's disease. It is rich in vitamins B6, C, K, niacin, thiamine, and various minerals like phosphorus, zinc, potassium, magnesium, and selenium. Zinc in the garlic helps immunity. It further has the potential to enhance gut and digestive health, which adds to overall well-being.

Incorporating raw garlic into the daily routine, especially on an empty stomach, would open up a world of several health benefits.

1. Immune support: Due to the allicin in raw garlic which has antimicrobial properties it would bolster the immune system, which would ward off infections and colds.

2. Heart health: Garlic contributes to lowering cholesterol and blood pressure. Eating it raw enhances cardiovascular benefits contributing to better heart health.

3. Digestive health: Garlic stimulates the digestive system by promoting the growth of good bacteria. On an empty stomach, it can help to prevent gastrointestinal problems.

4. Detoxification: Raw garlic supports liver function and helps the detoxification process, aiding to removal of toxins from the body.

5. Blood sugar levels: Garlic helps with insulin sensitivity and diabetes.

6. Weight management: Garlic regulates metabolism and instils fat burning to manage weight.

7. Garlic can repair broken bones faster.

When garlic juice is applied to the skin, it may help heal psoriasis, cold sores, and acne. Garlic is also beneficial for ear infections due to its antimicrobial properties.

One more magical thing about garlic is that due to its very high antioxidant properties, it can prevent stomach, liver, prostate, bladder, colon, and even lung cancer.

For maximum benefits, it is important to crush or chop the garlic pods and let them sit for a few minutes before taking them. This process helps to activate their health-promoting compounds.

All in all, garlic has innumerable healing and system-regulating properties. I am sorry to say that not including it in your daily diet and not having it in its raw form reflects ignorance and disregard for the good things life and nature have to offer.

However, people with gastrointestinal problems should consult a healthcare professional before making any significant dietary changes.

The traditional Indian ceremony of applying haldi paste - the golden powder (turmeric) to the face, hands, and feet of would-be brides and grooms is a ritual as old as the hills.

The benefits of consuming turmeric internally and applying turmeric externally are endless and have been known for centuries.

CHAPTER 35

TURMERIC (CURCUMIN)

India was the first to discover the importance of turmeric to mankind. It has been exporting turmeric since ancient times to the world. It was known as the golden era.

Turmeric powder is derived from the root of the Curcuma longa plant. It is well known for its anti-inflammatory and antioxidant properties, primarily attributed to its active compound, curcumin.

When consumed, turmeric powder can support digestive function, enhance joint health, and bolster the immune system. Turmeric has been linked to much-improved brain function.

Its ability to fight oxidative stress would also play a role in reducing the risk of chronic heart diseases and cancer. Turmeric is known to combat metabolic syndrome.

Turmeric contains many useful compounds, but the best healing and health-giving compound in it is curcumin. It is the curcumin in turmeric that gives it that distinctive flavour, colour, and its efficacy to heal. In the world of Ayurveda, turmeric is wildly popular due to the power of the curcumin in it. Curcumin manages and reduces pain and inflammation in all forms of arthritis, including rheumatoid and osteoarthritis.

Topical direct application of curcumin quickly heals skin lacerations, cuts, bruises, and all open wounds. Turmeric studies have shown it has immense bifunctional properties that heal all wounds. It is also known as a primitive and deep scavenger of wounds. When applied to the skin, its antimicrobial and anti-inflammatory properties make it effective in reducing redness and skin irritation, including acne. It is also known to brighten the complexion and even out the tone of the skin. It is the best healer compared to all the medicated ointments and healing creams manufactured to date.

Many individuals use turmeric masks.

Turmeric and curcumin can both be effective against joint pains and bacterial and fungal infections. They contain the most effective supplements, antioxidants, and anti-inflammatory properties. Turmeric keeps all the blood vessels clean and clear of fat deposits. It enhances good blood flow.

CHAPTER 36

ASHWAGANDHA OH, TO BE YOUNG AGAIN

Ashwagandha, the Indian Ginseng, is one of the oldest known herbs in Ayurveda.

With the advent of new scientific research, there is renewed interest in Ashwagandha, and it is gaining popularity once again. The latest findings have revealed amazing all-round benefits of Ashwagandha. This magnificent herb is also used to avoid premature ageing.

Ashwagandha builds a very substantial and healthy immune system to regulate and sustain overall health. It builds a perfect defence mechanism to help create infection-fighting cells, thus shielding your body from most infections.

Ashwagandha improves brain function and works wonders on memory. Its antioxidant properties protect the brain cells from harmful free radicals, which keep the brain in peak health well into very late age.

Ashwagandha or Ginseng are usually used as adaptogens, which are roots and herbs of non-toxic plants that help the body resist stress of all kinds: physical, biological, and chemical. This extract helps the body's ability to resist the damaging effects of long-term complications. For this reason, Ashwagandha is known to be a great stress buster. It has compounds that can calm the mind, help moods, relieve stress, and help fight physical and mental duress. It is very beneficial in fighting insomnia and supporting restful sleep.

Ashwagandha lowers blood pressure and improves the immune system. Due to its anti-inflammatory properties, it relieves pain all the way to the central nervous system. It helps to strengthen the nervous system. It improves heart health by reducing the bad cholesterol and triglycerides. It increases insulin secretion and helps in reducing sugar levels.

Latest research has shown that Ashwagandha is a very potent root that can fight cancer. It can induce the death of pre-existing cancer cells and reduce the growth of new cells.

For men, Ashwagandha boosts their testosterone levels, increases sperm count, enhances sexual desire, and improves erectile dysfunction.

For women, Ashwagandha enhances fertility and menstrual health. It helps increase blood flow and reduces sexual dysfunction. It increases libido in men and women, promotes sexual desire, and increases sexual performance.

To conclude, let me emphasise that Ashwagandha is known for its adaptogenic attributes, helping the body to manage anxiety and stress. Moreover, it would improve focus and support overall well-being by balancing cortisol levels and promoting better, deeper sleep. The final results make you feel years younger in many ways.

CHAPTER 37

NUTS

1. **Almonds:**

"Akkal badam khanay se nahi milti hain. akkal dokha khanay se milti hain!"

"You do not become smart by eating almonds. You get smart after being betrayed."

But almonds do sharpen the mind and memory. Almonds improve brain function.

While most people consider almonds as nuts, they are seeds enclosed in the fruit of an almond tree. Almonds are rich in antioxidants and nutrients such as proteins, fibre, vitamin E, potassium, zinc, vitamin K, calcium, magnesium, and phosphorus. They are considered the perfect food.

Almonds strengthen the bones and teeth because of its high calcium content. It lowers blood sugar levels, as well as bad cholesterol, and brings the blood pressure down. They contain a lot of good, healthy, monounsaturated, and polyunsaturated fats, which have a positive impact on the heart as well as on brain health.

Finally, roasted almonds are a very delicious and healthy snack. Consuming six or seven almonds daily has immense nutritional benefits.

2. **Walnuts:**

Walnuts overflow with nature's best nutrients. They are low in saturated fats, trans fats, and sodium. They contain vitamins A and C, fibre, proteins, and an abundance of calcium and iron. They are brimming with healthy, unsaturated omega-3 fatty acids.

It is known as the heart-and-brain-healthy food for children, adults, and aged seniors. Walnuts boost memory, moods, and the functioning of the brain. From heart health to the brain cells, it enhances mental health. Latest studies show that it increases the good cholesterol HDL and lowers the bad cholesterol LDL. Walnuts contain polyphenols, which help the digestive system and go a long way in improving gut health.

Consuming two or three whole walnuts a day gives their full benefit.

3. **Pistachios:**

Like almonds, pistachios are called nuts but are actually seeds. To eat the seed, you have to crack open the outer shell.

Among all other nuts, pistachios have the highest protein content. Pistachios have a high calorie-to-protein ratio, so consuming them fills you up very quickly, and you will not feel hungry. They are good for decreasing your weight and your waistline.

Due to their high fibre content and high monounsaturated and polyunsaturated fat content, they protect you from the risk of heart disease and control your cholesterol levels. Pistachios can help maintain your blood pressure. They promote healthy gut bacteria and, being probiotic in nature, they help digestion.

Pistachios have a low glycaemic index, phenolic compounds, and antioxidants which maintain the sugar levels in your system. They are not only a very tasty snack, but also a very healthy snack. One can buy pistachios in various forms: shelled, unshelled, roasted, honeyed, or salted.

4. **Peanuts:**

Peanuts do not meet the botanical standards of a true nut. They are legumes and are formed like peas in a pod.

Peanuts are replete in protein content and are rich in vitamins C and E, copper, magnesium, phosphorus, and different plant compounds that are beneficial to our health. Vitamin C and E give additional elasticity to our skin. Other known nutrients of the peanut are niacin and vitamin B1, which keep dementia and Alzheimer's at bay as we age. They have polyunsaturated and monounsaturated fats that are good for the body. They are devoid of trans fats that are harmful to the body.

Peanuts help support the bones, maintaining a healthy skeletal system. Thus, these vitamins, compounds, and nutrients help strengthen our bones for old age.

Peanuts are rich in resveratrol, which delays our ageing, prevents early wrinkles on our hands and face, and helps to keep eczema and psoriasis in check. Peanuts have a very high satiety. They fill one up and prevent overeating by satiating hunger.

However, peanuts are often short-changed and described as the poor man's snack. They are a good and very affordable substitute for cashews, almonds, and pistachios.

Peanuts are often used with drinks due to their mouth-watering, crunchy taste and don't leave a hole in your purse. They are very popular, easily available, and affordable snack.

With a drink in hand and peanuts on the table, let us salute the little nut. Cheers!!

5. **Cashew nuts:**

Cashew nuts are considered the king of all nuts.

These tiny kidney-shaped nuts are usually grown in tropical climates. Cashew nuts contain a range of minerals, vitamins, plant compounds, fibre, and healthy fats. They are packed with nutrients and heart-healthy fats. However, cashew nuts contain a lot of saturated fats and should not be eaten in excess.

Cashews are abundant in good fats and are free from cholesterol. Their rich nutrients keep the heart healthy. They are filled with proanthocyanins and copper, which prevent the cancerous growth of tumour cells in the body. That is one of the lesser-known advantages of eating cashew nuts every day.

Another lesser-known fact is that the lutein that cashew nuts contain, along with other antioxidants, promotes healthy eyesight. Due to the taste of cashew nuts, they are the number one choice for a snack. If a plate full of mixed nuts is laid out, cashews are the first to get over. They are a treat on the tongue. However, it is not something you can binge on. Having five or six cashews every day is preferable and good for cholesterol levels.

6. **Other nuts:**

Hazelnuts, chestnuts, macadamia nuts, Brazil nuts, pine nuts, pecan nuts, and many more fall under the category of nuts. Most nuts have numerous health benefits; they protect the heart, bones, and muscles, and potentially also against cancer. Many are very appealing to our taste buds.

Delicious, delectable, and full of different and delightful flavours, these various nuts appeal to our taste buds. Tasty, yummy, appetising, scrumptious, and mouth-watering are some of the adjectives to describe them.

CHAPTER
38

MORINGA, THE MAGIC PLANT

The Moringa tree, a native plant of India, is often known as the "miracle tree of life" due to its impressive nutritional value and health-giving properties. It has been known for centuries for its healing properties.

However, until recently, very little was known about the varied richness of this magical plant. New research has recognised it for its medicinal value, and it is now one of the most powerful herbal supplements. True to its given name as the miracle tree, the bark, leaves, seeds, and roots of the moringa tree are beneficial to mankind.

Here are some reasons for its reputation.

Antimicrobial properties: it is found to have anti fungal and antibacterial properties, which fight off infections.

The moringa leaves, when dried and powdered, are an excellent source of multiple vitamins such as B2, B3 (Riboflavin and Niacin), folate, and B6, vitamins A and C, together with Omega-3 fatty acids. They also contain a very high percentage of plant-based proteins, calcium, and potassium for muscle and bone building, and essential amino acids.

Being rich in fibre, it is a great aid in digestion. It prevents the formation and restricts the invasion of bad bacteria and pathogens due to its anti-inflammatory properties. It flushes out unhealthy toxins and clears waste products from the system. It is like an army of soldiers protecting our guts.

The Moringa plant has a plethora of antioxidants, which can fight oxidative stress in the body. It contains beta-carotene, a compound that regenerates healthy cell growth, repairs cell damage, and prevents premature ageing. This delays the formation of premature wrinkling of the skin.

The plant further contains a rich source of iron and magnesium, which helps blood circulation and the flow of oxygenated blood to the entire body. This brings enough blood to help the optimum functioning of the brain.

Moringa powder has antiseptic and antimicrobial properties that help in healing. It works as an antibiotic and fights any viral infection. When added to the diet, it energises and strengthens you to fight any weakness, fatigue, and debility that comes your way.

It brings down bad LDL levels, which is good for heart health. It also brings down sugar levels in patients suffering from type 2 diabetes.

Since moringa contains all these nutritionally rich ingredients, it makes you more spirited and dynamic, supports your moods, and enhances cognition.

Moringa is an affordable alternative medicine and is fast becoming a low-priced superfood. It can be ingested as tablets or in powder form. Though it may sound unbelievable, within a few weeks, you will notice a marked difference in your overall health.

Moringa can be a great supplement, but it should not replace a balanced diet rich in various nutrients. Consuming the Moringa plant has no side effects. However, some individuals may experience digestive or allergic issues. It is better to monitor your body's response.

A word of caution: While it is good for constipation, Moringa taken in excess can have a laxative effect. Start slow, with a teaspoon or two daily.

In summary, moringa can be a very beneficial addition to your list of herbs in your diet, but it is best to consult your healthcare provider if you plan to take it daily.

However, my family and I have been taking moringa for a long time, and the difference it has made to our health is amazing. Besides, it is an unbeatable value for money.

May I add here that it is one of the lowest-cost options to revive and revamp your health in a short period of time.

It is widely available online. So what are you, my dear reader, waiting for?

CHAPTER
39

CLOVE

Have you ever wondered if a simple kitchen spice can transform your body? Well, after 50, your body needs a little extra care. And guess what? Cloves might be the secret weapon you didn't know you needed. Packed with powerful antioxidants, anti-inflammatory properties, and essential nutrients, just two cloves a day could make a huge difference to your health.

Here's what will happen if you add cloves to your daily routine. It will boost your immune system like never before. As we age, our immune system naturally weakens, making it more susceptible to illnesses and infections. But cloves are rich in vitamin C, which can strengthen our body's defence system.

Cloves, along with cinnamon, are one of the main spices used in any Indian cuisine. They are used to flavour a large variety of spicy and savoury dishes, and sweet dishes. This flavourful, piquant, peppery, and aromatic spice is rich in healing properties. However, because of its spicy and slightly pungent flavour, it should be used sparingly in cooking and seasoning.

Back in the day, cloves or clove oil were used to prevent oral infections. Today, cloves are used to relieve toothaches by temporarily deadening the nerves in the affected portion of the gums. Along with pain-relieving properties, they help to eliminate plaque, gingivitis, and, of course, bad breath. Chewing one or two cloves a day prevents tooth decay. Chewing them before bedtime helps avoid oral infections. They can also be used as a mouth freshener.

Other ways of ingesting cloves are to soak two or three cloves in half a glass of water overnight and drink it in the morning on an empty stomach. Alternatively, you can boil two or three cloves in some water for a few minutes, then let it simmer. Drink it at room temperature before your meal. Clove water helps reduce body weight. Clove water also helps patients with arthritis.

Clove water is a great drink for your digestive system. It mixes with your saliva and increases the flow of gastric juices. This, in turn, relieves pain and indigestion and prevents gas formation. Cloves reduce digestive issues and inflammation.

Gently sucking on a clove that is held between your clenched teeth can ease breathing.

Cloves contain eugenol, which is most effective against harmful bacteria and fungal infections. However, limit your clove intake to two or three maximum a day. Overdosing on eugenol can be harmful in the long run and could affect the liver.

Cloves contain anti-carcinogenic properties, which can reduce the chances of lung, breast, and ovarian cancers. They give a boost to our immunity. Cloves are known to regulate blood sugar levels.

Cloves contain nutrients, anti-inflammatory agents, and antioxidants that strengthen and help the growth of hair.

To summarise, I would say eating a clove or two a day can offer several health benefits and medicinal properties.

1. Digestive health: Cloves aid in digestion. Reduce distention and gas.

2. Antioxidant properties: Reduces oxidative stress and reduces inflammation in the body.

3. Antimicrobial activity: Cloves have natural antimicrobial properties that help fight fungi and bacteria, healing oral health.

4. One or two cloves support liver function and prevent damage to the liver.

5. Respiratory health: Clove oil is often used to smoothen the respiratory tract and relieve cough.

6. Pain relief: Clove oil is often used to relieve toothache and dental care due to its analgesic effects.

7. Blood sugar regulation: It is well known that cloves can help regulate blood sugar levels. Managing sugar sensitivities a bit better.

Consuming cloves in moderation, i.e., two a day, is generally safe for most people.

A sweet and bitter juice that helps to reduce sugar in the blood.

CHAPTER 40

PANEER DODA/PHOOL

Paneer Doda Phool is known as the flower of the paneer plant. It has been traditionally valued for its potential health benefits, mainly for people trying to manage diabetes type 2.

The best way to ingest it is to soak the flowers in water overnight.

Soaking the flowers nightlong helps to increase their wholesomeness and enhance their beneficial properties and also makes them easier to digest.

For diabetics, the consumption of Paneer Doda Phool can help regulate blood sugar levels due to its low glycemic value index.

Furthermore, it is rich in fiber and antioxidants, which can help and assist in improving insulin sensitivity and can boost better digestive well being. The presence of essential minerals and vitamins in it also supports overall good health and state of being, making it a favourable supplement to a diabetic-helpful diet plan.

Regular use of the Paneer Doda Phool may contribute to better blood glucose control and reduce the risk of diabetes-related complexities.

A native plant of India, Pakistan, and Afghanistan, Paneer Doda/Phool (also known as *Indian Rennet* or by its Ayurvedic name, *Withania Coagulans*) is an excellent remedy to control blood sugar in patients with type 2 diabetes. While it does not cure diabetes, it does help you gain control over the sugar levels in your blood by aiding the utilisation of carbohydrates in the body. It also helps with liver function and reduces bad cholesterol.

To use Paneer Doda/Phool, soak five to six phools (flowers). If you are borderline diabetic or 8 to 10 phools if you are a severe diabetic, in a glass of water overnight. Squeeze the flowers in the morning or any time during the day, strain, and drink on an empty stomach.

No side effects have been reported in consuming Doda Phools, and it has not shown any negative interactions with other medications. Alternative herbal and Ayurveda products should not replace already prescribed medication by your doctor. It is advisable to consult your healthcare provider before making any changes. Many of these alternative remedies have been used by my family, close friends, and associates with excellent results.

However, there is not sufficient evidence that it is safe for pregnant and breastfeeding mothers and is therefore not recommended for this group.

—— CHAPTER ——
41

MELATONIN

In the olden days when we slept, we gave rest to our bodies. Today when we sleep we give rest to our mobile phones.

Sleep is absolutely essential for our body, mind, and soul. The rest we get, while we sleep, helps to regenerate the cells in our body, which is why adequate sleep is as important as the oxygen we breathe and as important as the food and water we need to sustain ourselves.

Most living beings have an internal 24-hour clock. That internal biological rhythm regulates the timing of our sleep patterns, and also our day and night cycles. Many of us will, at some point in our lives, struggle to get a few hours of natural sleep—a point when we don't get the much-required sleep we need; when we toss and turn for hours in bed. But sleep eludes us.

When we suffer from a long and severe break in our sleeping pattern, it is called insomnia. We are often driven to take some form of sleep medication. However, sleeping pills never resolve the problem. It is habit-forming and gradually, we need more and more sleep medication to get the recommended seven to nine hours of undisturbed sleep. This situation is harmful in the long run.

However, thanks to Mother Nature, our body produces and secretes a natural compound called melatonin. The pineal gland in our brain releases melatonin, which induces natural sleep. Melatonin has very positive effects on our brain. It does restorative work for the formation of new brain cells and improves long-term memory.

Melatonin is a hormone produced by the pineal gland in our brain, playing a very essential role in our sleep-wake pattern. Its production is influenced by the exposure to light. Darkness promotes melatonin secretion, which encourages sleep. Light inhibits our sleep. This natural day-night pattern synchronises our body clock, leading to a much-improved sleep pattern and improved sleep quality, which ensures our well-being, due to natural wear and tear.

Nature produces less melatonin during daylight. However, as the late evening approaches, production increases. Melatonin secretion is a natural process, but it is also found in man-made oral capsules and pills, which release the same melatonin. Melatonin is available at most online stores in 2 mg, 5 mg, 10 mg, and even 20 mg strengths.

Start with a low dosage. Take melatonin about half an hour before your bedtime and switch off all the bedroom lights. If you use a dim light in some corner of your room, keep it away from your eyes for a calmer, better, and longer sleep. In order to get the full effects of melatonin, sleep in a comfortable, cool, dark space or use an eye mask. Total darkness will give you a deep and restful sleep.

As a supplement, melatonin is often used to alleviate insomnia and jet lag, making it a popular choice for airline crew who work at odd hours in changing time zones.

Nature's ability to self-produce the hormone melatonin highlights the deep connection between bodily functions and the environment around us. Nature helps us to balance our day-night sleep patterns, thanks to natural light and dark patterns around us, maintaining our in-built 24-hour biological body cycle.

Melatonin is not recommended for long-term use. If your insomnia persists, it is advisable to see your medical practitioner.

Melatonin content and its secretion decrease as we age, and that is the reason we sleep less as we age. Also, lesser melatonin release is found in patients suffering from dementia, Alzheimer's, and diabetes.

I wish you, my dear reader, a very good night's sleep tonight, tomorrow night, and all the nights to come. I wish you many happy and sweet dreams. May all your dreams be fulfilled. Amen!

CHAPTER 42

KOKUM BUTTER

Kokum (Amsol) butter, native to India, is also known as Garcinia indica or Goa butter. It is a hardened oil made from the seeds of the fruit-bearing Kokum tree. The fruit and the seeds of this tree are used in a variety of cosmetic, culinary, and medicinal applications. It is a powerhouse of antioxidants and complex vitamins.

At room temperature, unrefined Kokum butter is hard and solid like a potato. It is beige or light brown, whereas the refined Kokum is white.

On the culinary front, Kokum butter is used in cooking for its distinctive flavour. With its sour taste, it is used in place of tamarind in South Indian cuisine, especially in curries. Kokum is also known as Malabar tamarind and is extensively used in Kerala, Maharashtra, and Konkani dishes.

For its cosmetic value, Kokum butter is a rich emollient. It hydrates and restores moisture to nourish and soften dry skin, cracked heels, dry hair, chapped lips, and the scalp.

It is the best healer for cracked heels. Heat the Kokum butter gently and apply the melted paste onto your cracked heels. It will get absorbed into the skin and heal the cracks like magic.

Kokum butter can soften and moisten any skin type and tone, from oily, dry, very dry, sensitive, acne-prone, or ageing skin, turning it glowing and glossy in a quick time. When applied to the skin, Kokum has very powerful moisturising properties. Due to its low comedogenic rating of less than 2, it does not clog the pores or cause any breakouts. This makes it a very safe ingredient to use on the face. In comparison, coconut oil has a very high comedogenic rating, which means its application blocks pores. As a result, coconut oil can make acne worse for some people and is not recommended for people with oily skin.

All these magical properties make Kokum butter highly sought after commercially in the cosmetic industry. It is used as an important ingredient in the manufacture of face creams, body lotions, lip balms, shampoos, soaps, hair oils, etc. However, applying the original and natural (refined or otherwise) Kokum butter directly without any other added ingredients to the skin has shown much better results than most creams and moisturisers sold in the market.

I stand by it and I swear by it! It also happens to be the cheapest value-for-money moisturising cream in the market. Go for it!

Millet is good for animals, great for birds, and exceptionally marvellous for humans.

Let us not undervalue the role of the little millet.

CHAPTER 43

MILLETS

Millet crops are a family of cereal crops like grains. They come in two categories: small and large, and they belong to the grass family Poaceae. Millets are cultivated in Asia and Africa. India is the largest producer of millets in the world, and it produces 75% of the millets grown in all of Asia. This year has been declared as the International Year of Millet, in order to promote more awareness, production, and consumption of the crop.

Millets are plants with a lot of tiny seeds in leafy folds that are used to cook a variety of different foods. They have a great advantage over most other crops because they are pest- and climate-resistant. They adapt to any unfavourable conditions. They can survive in drought-ridden, minimally fertile soil and harsh environments. Millets usually require less water but can also thrive in excessively heavy rains.

In most parts of the world, the maximum consumption has always been rice and wheat.

Rice is a good source of energy, but it contains a high percentage of simple carbohydrates. Consuming white rice (also known as polished rice) brings on weight gain and may lead to obesity. Rice, where the bran and germ layers are not removed and polished off, leaves a brown shade and is called brown rice. This rice is a much healthier variety. Brown rice prevents obesity and also controls sugar levels in the blood. It is good for diabetics.

However, millets are a better and healthier option. Millets have more calories, fibre, and good fat, more proteins, minerals, and vitamins. Millets have a much lower glycemic index than wheat. They provide far superior nutrient density, cause less of insulin spike in the blood, and contain more dietary fibre. Traditionally, millets are consumed as a staple diet in rural India. Millets are popularly known as a poor man's diet.

All millets have very high nutritional value and contain exceptional health benefits. Millets are a great source of plant compounds, essential minerals, vitamin B, antioxidants, calcium, zinc, high in protein, iron, and fibre content. They are also high in carbs.

Millets boost our immune system and fight free radicals in the body. They are also gluten-free. Even gluten-sensitive individuals with celiac disease can enjoy their benefits.

In all, millets are good all around: for the heart, for cholesterol, for sugar levels, for the nervous system, and for the gut.

There is a long list of different varieties of millet grown in Asia and Africa, but there are only a few varieties that are popular and widely consumed in India. All of them provide very good nutrient value. They can all be cooked in various ways, in different cuisines, and are easy to digest. Consumed more in rural India, some of the popular names in Hindi are Bajra, Kangana, Jowar, Ragi, Kulthi dal, and Chana.

Here are the benefits:

Pearl millet (Bajra)

Pearl millet boosts bowel movement and increases energy levels. It also relaxes the body and fights insomnia.

Foxtail millets (Kangana)

Foxtail millets are high in calcium and iron. They are traditionally used for children due to easy absorption and digestion. They can cure anaemia.

Sorghum millet (Jowar)

Sorghum millets improve digestive health. Their high fibre content increases the good cholesterol and brings down the bad cholesterol, enhancing heart health.

Finger millet (Ragi)

Finger millets are a very important source of natural iron and calcium. They help patients with anaemia and build strong bones. They are very beneficial for the old as well as growing children.

Horse gram (Kulthi dal)

Horse gram is a very rich source of proteins and fibre and is good for digestive health. It also reduces blood sugar by reducing insulin resistance.

Proso millets (Chenna)

Proso millets are an excellent source of lecithin, which builds a strong functioning nervous system.

Eating millet offers numerous health benefits, including improved digestion, potential support for heart health, and high nutritional value, making them a great addition to our diet.

CHAPTER
44

MILK THISTLE

We usually worry about the condition of our heart, our brain, kidneys, and lungs. They are vital to our health. But how many of us know that our liver is equally important for our bodies to function normally? More than two million people in the world succumb to liver diseases every year.

Milk thistle is derived from a Silybum Marianum plant which contains silymarin, a compound that is rich in anti-inflammatory and antioxidant properties. Regular intake of milk thistle helps improve conditions like fatty liver and even liver cirrhosis. Research indicates that milk thistle can potentially improve liver enzyme levels and provide overall liver health.

Milk thistle can support liver health but is not a cure and should not replace conventional medications.

Milk thistle is a supplement that has been used for years in Ayurveda. It has been used to help and improve fatty liver, cirrhosis, jaundice, hepatitis, and all pathological problems concerning the liver. It is very vital for the proper functioning of our liver and even our gall bladder. An ingredient in the plant known as silymarin is effective in avoiding the toxicity of the liver. Silymarin is known to protect the liver from toxins.

One of the many reasons for liver problems and, ultimately, liver diseases is excessive alcohol consumption. Uncontrolled drinking every day over the years usually leads to fatty liver and then to cirrhosis of the liver. Other causes that lead to fatty liver could be obesity, high blood sugar levels, blood pressure, cholesterol, and triglycerides. However, a large percentage of the two million deaths are attributed to heavy consumption of alcohol.

People with liver damage would want to know if their liver will heal if they quit drinking. The answer to that is both yes and no. Healing can begin a few weeks after stopping alcohol consumption. But depending on the extent of damage to the liver, it may or may not heal fully. The liver is one of the few organs in our body that does not regenerate itself very easily.

Each time the liver filters the alcohol in the system, some of the cells in the liver die. The immune system in the body can and does regenerate the cells, but over a period of time, the cells lose their ability to regenerate. If a large percentage of the liver is damaged due to misuse of alcohol or certain medications, toxins, and viruses, then it scars the liver. This scarring of tissues in the liver over a period of time would probably result in cirrhosis of the liver.

Jaundice is another problem that occurs due to a damaged liver. Signs of jaundice are yellowing of the skin and the eyes. Nausea and vomiting are accompanied by dark yellow urine output.

Fortunately, milk thistle can reverse the damage to the liver to a great extent.

Milk thistle supplements in the form of capsules are available in all online and medical stores. One capsule taken orally two or three times daily may help to reverse the damage.

Besides Milk Thistle, Ayurveda also has a product named Liv 52 which helps the liver.

Indian Ginseng, i.e., Ashwagandha, and raw garlic are good for the liver to function properly.

Another very active compound, glycyrrhizin, is found in the extract from the liquorice root. Liquorice root is like candy. It has antiviral, anti-inflammatory, and many other liver-protecting properties. Chinese and Japanese traditionally use glycyrrhizin for most liver ailments.

Whether you drink alcohol or not, it is a good idea to include the liver profile test in your half-yearly health check-up.

Remember, *Life depends on the Liver.*

CHAPTER 45

GARCINIA CAMBOGIA

Garcinia Cambogia is a pumpkin-like, greenish-yellow coloured fruit that is native to Southeast Asia and found widely in India.

The peel of the fruit contains a plant compound hydroxycitric acid (HCA) which suppresses your appetite and prevents fat production by blocking an enzyme called citrate lyase, which the body uses to transform carbohydrates into fat. It is a very well-known and prevalent weight loss supplement. Besides weight loss, it also reduces the fat around the belly in people who are overweight and obese.

Garcinia Cambogia is known for its ability to lose weight, particularly when accompanied by a healthy diet, regular physical activity, and/or regular exercise. While most people would experience weight loss, it is important to approach it as a supplement to a well-balanced lifestyle, rather than a solitary cure-all solution.

It reduces the torments of hunger by augmenting the serotonin levels in the brain. Serotonin is also a mood booster. An increase in serotonin levels stabilises moods and the happiness quotient. A lack of serotonin results in anxiety and depression.

For the Garcinia Cambogia supplement to be most effective, it should be taken about one hour before meals. To reap maximum benefits, mix it with apple cider vinegar in a glass of water and consume it 30 to 60 minutes before meals twice a day. Adding a bit of ginger and cinnamon to the mixture enhances the taste and improves the digestive process further.

Garcinia reduces the fat in your blood and the oxidative stress in your body. However, Garcinia Cambogia is definitely not recommended for long-term use. Neither are people who have liver problems like jaundice, fatty liver, etc. If taken for the long term or exceeding the recommended dosage, it can result in liver damage.

Do not exceed the time frame or dosage recommended on the bottle.

As always, please consult your doctor before starting on Garcinia Cambogia, as with most herbal medicines. Besides, one should not partake in it for the long term.

CHAPTER

46

AMLA

Amla, a super fruit, is known as the divine fruit from heaven. Surprisingly, it is not given the credit it deserves. It is a remarkably beneficial medicinal plant that is native to Asia and is very popular all over India for medicinal preparations in Ayurveda. Ancient sages and Rishis described Amla as a fruit with anti-ageing properties, known for boosting overall immunity and metabolism.

Amla has a rich concentration of vitamin C compared to all other fruits. It is rich in flavonoids, vitamins A and B, fibre, carotene, calcium, and minerals. It has excellent anti-inflammatory, antibacterial, immunity-strengthening, and antioxidant properties.

Amla is one of the best for rejuvenation of the whole body. It is good for your heart, lungs, blood, liver, skin, and bones.

Amla has several benefits for the skin. It makes your skin look and feel younger. Amla juice is a natural blood cleanser and purifier and prevents acne, pimples, and pigmentation. If amla is applied directly, it lightens the skin marks, brightens, and moisturises dry skin. Like collagen, it contributes to the firmness as well as softness of the skin.

Amla improves hair growth, repairs hair follicles, and prevents dandruff and dryness. Most herbal hair products use

Amla as an ingredient to prevent hair loss and make the hair thicker, shinier, and softer to the touch.

Amla helps prevent cancer and also improves our memory.

Amla has a very unique taste. It is bitter, sour, and sweetly pungent too. It is used in India for various culinary purposes, from pickles, murabbas (sweet pickles), and sweet and sour chutneys to main dishes as well.

To summarise, the Indian gooseberry has several health benefits.

1. Improves digestion.

2. Supports heart health.

3. Rich in vitamins A, B, C, and many minerals.

4. Improves skin, scalp, and hair health.

5. Regulates blood sugar levels.

6. Enhances digestion.

7. Boosts immunity.

8. Rich in antioxidants.

9. Combats ageing.

The Indian gooseberry or Amla is packed with super nutrients. It is rich in vitamin C and is considered a top-quality, prime food.

Strangely, the goodness of Amla is not widely known, nor broadly used.

Be smart. Buy Amla today.

There never was, and never will be a healthier fruit.

CHAPTER 47

AVOCADOS

We have all grown up with "*An apple a day keeps the doctor away.*"

However, I say, "An avocado a day will keep the doctor away."

The benefits of this fruit are many. Too many to count. You name it, the avocado has it. No wonder, it is hailed as the king of fruits due to its rich nutritional profile and many health-giving boons.

Healthy fat is essential for every cell in our body to support the immune system. Avocado provides a plethora of healthy and beneficial monounsaturated fatty acids. It contains healthy fats, fibre, bioactive compounds, and carotenoids. It increases the power of absorption of fat-soluble nutrients. It is packed with 20 minerals and vitamins A, C, D, E, and K are just some of them. Avocados are loaded with riboflavin, niacin, beta-carotene, magnesium, potassium, and Omega-3 fatty acids. In addition to high-quality fibre, avocado possesses phytochemicals and multiple nutrients. It lowers your blood pressure and reduces the risk of heart disease by increasing HDL levels (good cholesterol).

Kudos to vitamin A in the avocado—it brings back lost collagen to our skin. It has powerful anti-inflammatory compounds and antioxidants which keep our inner and outer skin glowing naturally and wrinkle-free.

Avocados are a great source of folate, which negates the production of homocysteine, an amino acid that lessens the flow of healthy nutrients to the brain. High homocysteine levels damage the insides of our arteries and increase the risk of blood clots, heart disease, stroke, and dementia. Nature has blessed us with a fruit that will not only nullify but annihilate all these negative complications.

Moreover, avocados are innumerably versatile in their culinary attributes. Enhancing various dishes with their subtle flavour and creamy texture. Their combination of health rewards and culinary adaptability solidifies the reputation of the avocado as the king of fruits and a unique blend of a powerhouse of good health.

If you can't add one full avocado to your diet every day, at least add half an avocado to take advantage of the fruits of this awesome fruit.

In conclusion, avocados are a powerhouse of nutrients, offering healthy fats that support skin health, promote heart health, provide crucial vitamins and antioxidants, and improve overall well-being. Making them additionally a delightful supplement to your diet.

CHAPTER 48

CINNAMON

Cinnamon is a spice that comes from the inner bark of a tree that belongs to the Cinnamomum family. It has been known for hundreds of years. The inner bark of the tree can be rolled into small sticks or ground into powder, which is used in various cuisines and baking. Thanks to its many beneficial compounds, cinnamon is associated with many health benefits.

There are two types of cinnamon: Cassia and Ceylon cinnamon. Cassia cinnamon contains a plant chemical called coumarin, which, if taken in large doses, could be harmful to the liver. The Cassia cinnamon should be avoided. The Ceylon variety is known as the true Cinnamon since it contains only traces of coumarin.

Cinnamon is a powerhouse of antioxidants. It can prevent type 2 diabetes. But if a person is already diabetic, cinnamon helps to block the enzyme that aids glucose absorption in the blood. This way, it can manage diabetes by lowering blood sugar.

Cinnamon is good for the heart because it helps to reduce the bad cholesterol (LDL) and may increase the good cholesterol (HDL). It neutralises free radicals in the body, thereby protecting the body's cells from damage and oxidative stress, further reducing the chances of heart-related ailments.

Cinnamon is loaded with antioxidants that protect against inflammation, disease, and ageing. It also has antibacterial properties that prevent mouth infections and bad breath.

Cinnamon kills bacteria in the gut that infect the intestines and cause bloating, stomach pains, and dysentery, resulting in IBS.

Last but not least, cinnamon helps fight cancer. It protects the DNA and, in turn, prevents the growth of tumours that could turn cancerous. It contains a compound called Cinnamaldehyde which inhibits the growth of tumours in the body.

With all these benefits, it is a good idea to take cinnamon powder or cinnamon supplements daily in small amounts as directed on the bottle. These supplements are concentrated to deliver a very specific dose of the essential oils of this herb as well as other related plant compounds.

Cinnamon can be a healthy ingredient in your diet when consumed in moderation. It has several health benefits, including:

1. Antimicrobial properties

2. Heart health

3. Blood sugar control

4. Antioxidant properties

5. Anti-inflammatory effects

However, it is important to note that taking too much if you are already on medication for diabetes, liver, or heart disease is not advisable. Consuming it in moderation daily can be beneficial, but it is best to stick to the recommended minimal dosage in order to avoid any potential adverse effects. Especially with the cassia cinnamon, which contains higher levels of coumarin.

It is best to consume cinnamon as a spice in food as part of a balanced diet.

Red chillies/Cayenne, fresh or in its supplement form, are one of the last but not the least, God's gift to mankind.

CHAPTER 49

CAYENNE (RED CHILLIES)

Eating cayenne or red chillies, fresh or dried daily can have a multitude of health benefits, mainly due to their active compound, capsaicin, which is responsible for their spiced flavour and the heat in the chillies.

It is this compound that goes a long way in triggering positive effects on our cardiovascular health. Cayenne produces excellent flexibility and eases the blood flow to all our blood vessels, boosting the blood circulation in our body.

This compound, capsaicin, improves blood vessel function by enhancing endothelial health. By the way, endothelial health is the health of the inner lining of our blood vessels. Therefore, when the inner lining, i.e. endothelium, and lymphatic vessels are relaxed and open, the blood flows smoothly and keeps all body tasks functioning well.

The endothelium helps in the prevention of the formation of blood clots, further supporting vascular health. It also regulates inflammation and keeps toxins out.

Regular consumption of cayenne or red chillies (or their supplement form capsules) also helps to lower blood pressure, reduce bad cholesterol levels (LDL), and lower triglycerides in the system. While cayenne or red chillies can be beneficial to one's health, moderation is the key.

Here is a list of numerous health benefits of taking them whole or their supplements.

1. Supports digestive health: Cayenne stimulates the production of digestive enzymes which promotes gut health.

2. Improves blood circulation: Daily intake helps promote blood circulation by relaxing and dilating the blood vessels leading to more oxygen and better nutrient delivery throughout the body.

3. Improves heart health: Lowers blood pressure and bad cholesterol levels reducing the risk of heart disease. Its anti-inflammatory properties support cardiovascular health.

4. Supports digestive health: Cayenne or Red chillies can increase digestive enzymes by promoting healthy gut flora.

5. Boosts metabolism: Cayenne pepper contains capsaicin which can increase the metabolic rate and induce fat burning, which can aid in managing weight.

6. Boosts respiratory health: Cayenne gives relief from congestion and other respiratory issues helping to clear the mucus from the airways.

7. Pain relief: Fresh Cayenne is often used in pain relief ointments and creams to apply topically on the skin to relieve pain. These ointments have analgesic properties which give relief from pain.

8. Boosts immunity: Red chillies or Cayenne or its supplements have oxidation properties that fight stress which contributes to overall health.

While cayenne/red chillies or their supplement form have various benefits, few individuals may experience gastrointestinal irritation or discomfort. So it is good to start with smaller portions and fewer doses of the supplements, and then slowly increase it.

It is important to know that the smaller the chilli, the more potent and more pungent it will be.

CHAPTER
50

THE UNTOLD BENEFITS OF EGGS

What came first? The chicken or the egg?

A smart Parsi would reply, "Whatever was ordered first."

Since the time man has domesticated the chicken, eggs have been on breakfast menus in most countries of the world. Eggs are nutrient-rich, supplying almost every nutrient the body needs. Both the egg white and the yolk are rich in nutrients.

The yolk contains many minerals and vitamins, including vitamins A, B5, B12, D, E, zinc, calcium, selenium, and antioxidants. It is also rich in iron and Omega-3 fatty acids. The vitamins in the eggs support brain health and help the nervous system to function normally.

The white of the egg contains collagen, which fights inflammation and reduces wrinkles and fine lines, preventing the skin from early ageing.

Eggs are nature's premium protein food. They contain all nine essential amino acids required for growth and development. The high amount of leucine, an amino acid, in eggs helps muscle growth. The protein in eggs helps build strong muscles. A diet rich in eggs helps maintain body tissues and muscle growth. That is why wrestlers, bodybuilders, and weightlifters consume dozens of eggs daily. The rich protein comes from the egg white.

Eggs support the retina to function normally and also delay the deterioration of vision as one grows older.

In the recent past, theories were floated about the harmful effects of eggs. It was claimed that they increase LDL, the bad cholesterol, resulting in heart problems. However, that was a myth and remains a myth. Eggs are worth their weight in gold for the body.

Here is a list of the benefits of having eggs every day.

1. Eggs are nutrient-rich: Eggs are a rich source of proteins, vitamin D, B12, riboflavin, and minerals such as phosphorous and selenium.

2. Eggs contain healthy fat: They contain Omega-3 fatty acids which are good for heart health.

3. Eggs are good for long-term eye care: Eggs contain a rich supply of antioxidants like lutein, which is beneficial for eye health and prevents cataracts and eye degeneration.

4. Eggs are a good source of choline, which is important for brain health.

5. Aids weight management indirectly: Consuming eggs promotes a feeling of satiety and fullness.

6. LDL: Eggs contain large amounts of cholesterol. However, for most people dietary cholesterol has a much lesser impact on the body compared to trans fat and saturated fats.

Eggs are very versatile in any kitchen. From the head chef to the housewife, eggs are very flexible and adaptable and can be used with a variety of ingredients.

Finally, if I were to speak like a true Bawa, a Parsi, *"Sali Per Eedoo, Potatoes Per Eedoo, Bhaji Per Eedoo, Bhinda Per Eedoo, And Also Kheema (Mutton mince) Per Eedoo."*

"A couple of eggs with everything and anything under it would be the top of my menu, including the previous night's leftover cooked vegetable dishes. (meaning eggs on almost everything)." That would be a genuine Parsi breakfast.

CHAPTER
51

COLLAGEN PEPTIDES – THE FOUNTAIN OF YOUTH

If ever there was a fountain of youth, it would be collagen, collagen, and collagen.

Collagen is a supplement that will give the skin elasticity and hydration. It makes your skin smooth, supple, and wrinkle-free. The collagen in our skin helps heal all wounds rapidly, including the process of healing severe burns.

It makes your hair thicker, shinier, and stronger, and your nails, as they say, tough-as-nails. It also helps increase muscle mass.

Collagen supplements come in capsules, powder, and liquid form. Within four to six weeks of starting the supplement, you will see these improvements. It also plays a key role in maintaining and repairing your joints and your digestive tract.

Natural collagen in the body increases most significantly in infants, children, and young adults. It is at its peak in the early 20s. The production of collagen starts to drop with age, approximately 1.5% every year. By the time you are 60+, you have lost all the collagen in your body.

Chronological ageing shows on our skin, nails, and hair. As we age, the skin forms new fine lines and wrinkles. Our skin begins to loosen and sag. Our hair begins to thin, and our nails become brittle. We also begin to lose muscle and bone mass. In time, all this becomes increasingly visible.

As our bodies begin to stop the formation of new collagen, we can take collagen supplements orally to replenish our collagen peptides and amino acid levels. Collagen supplements strengthen and increase our bone density and the skeletal structure of our body. Adequate collagen in our bones goes a long way in decreasing the osteoarthritis pains in our joints.

Like so many health supplements, it is recommended that we take the required daily dosage with, before, or after our meals as shown on the label.

Here I would like to cite my own experiences about my battles with skin problems for several years.

I inherited very dry skin and psoriasis from the paternal side of my family. For years, I consulted with different skin specialists and dermatologists. I spent time inside infrared light machines and took a range of different medicines, creams, lotions, gels, and steroids. At best, these approaches would send my psoriasis into hibernation for some time. Then it would reappear with the slightest stress or sometimes for no reason.

A month's supply of collagen herbal powder did wonders for my skin. Gradually, my psoriasis got better and is almost non-existent now. My wife and I shall have it every day until our dying day.

I can now very proudly shout "Eureka!" I have found a permanent cure, thanks to collagen!

It was magic!

Today, I have forgotten that I ever had scars and scabs on my skin. This extraordinary herb can be the biggest blessing as we age.

CHAPTER 52

SAARO MAANAS: A GOOD MAN

My family has nicknamed me Saaro Maanas, meaning "a good man". Contrary to the meaning, the name was bestowed on me because, without exception, I believe and trust each and every one who comes into my life.

You can call me a humanist—I have faith in humanity, believe in the basic goodness of humans, and value each individual at face value. To this end, God has blessed me with all good people in my 83 years on this planet. To date, no one has broken my trust in them.

I neither preach nor do I teach anyone how to live their life. We have only one life, and everyone should live their life the way they want to. I do not profess to hold the secrets to a successful, happy, long, and fulfilled life.

I have lived a very charmed, happy, and fun-filled life. And within my limitations, I have had a very successful life so far. My very gratifying life started with the most wonderful and loving parents any child could ever hope to have.

My dearest, beloved mother, Jala Nader Sanjana, to me, was the most beautiful, angelic, admirable, kindest, and most devoted wife and mother that ever walked on Mother Earth. It is said that *God takes soonest those He loveth best*. God called my mother when she was only 55 years old. Her passing away was one of the saddest and most grief-stricken days of my life.

My dearest and most honourable father, Nader Jehangir Sanjana, was one of the strongest men India had seen in those days. He was a multiple gold and silver medallist wrestler. He was also a courageous and fearless shikari in his younger days. Hunting big cats in the 1920s and 30s was a sport during the British Raj. But he never killed for sport.

My father was very well-known as a saviour and a hero to the villagers of Castle Rock in Uttar Kannada. Scores of hapless villagers settled just outside the very dense forests in the Western Ghats, in Uttar Kannada, located in the state of Karnataka. They shared the forest with man-eating panthers and tigers. These man-eating wild cats would tread very stealthily, stalk the villagers (only humans, never the cattle!), surprise, attack, kill, and drag away the poor, half-alive victims from the villages close to the impenetrable jungles. My father would be called urgently by the Gram Panchayat to rid the village of these wild animals. It was his mission to make the village a safer place to live in.

My beloved mother became a victim of pleurisy (water formation in the lungs) which led to the third and fourth-stage cancer of her lungs.

Just a few years after my mother passed away, my father's health deteriorated very rapidly. In a case of *from the sublime to the ridiculous!* he underwent no fewer than four to five major heart attacks and survived. My father's cardiologist, Dr Farokh E. Udvada of Breach Candy Hospital, Bombay, said that in all his years of practicing medicine, my father was the only patient who survived five heart attacks.

Unfortunately, my father succumbed to his sixth major heart attack and passed away at the age of 64. My parents are now happy and healthy, and they walk with God Almighty! No more pain. No more aches.

My elder brother, Rusi, who is ten years older than me, has always been my mentor and my guiding light. He is one of the nicest brothers anyone can ever hope to have. I owe him a lot for whatever I am today.

My dearest sister, Lily, is my childhood companion and my best friend. Being four years older than me, she was also my protector and childhood guardian. Her getting married at the tender age of 17 and leaving our family home felt like the sun setting on a very cold winter evening. Although I was happy for Lily, I was temporarily heartbroken.

God has been very good to me. My wife Maloo and I have been happily married for the last 59 years. She has always been the love of my life. She gave me Zeena and Jennifer—two beautiful, compassionate, benevolent, humane, and wonderful daughters in the world. Ten sons could not have done better!

My two daughters gave us two very good-natured, handsome, successful, fabulous, and outstanding sons-in-law, Mehernosh and Serge, and three most awesome, loving, thoughtful, beautiful grandchildren—Kaizia, Kayan, and Gisele. What more can my wife and I ask for?

SAARO MAANAS: A GOOD MAN – THE MASTER KEY

As someone who has found and stayed in touch with most of my loving school friends from my early days at St. Xavier's School, Ahmedabad, in the mid-50s, and more than a thousand crew members, ex-colleagues, and friends from my working years at Air India since 1962, I can say I have a Master Key to love, life, and happiness!

Allow me to share it with my readers.

1. Speak no ill of anyone and only speak the good you know of everyone.

2. Eliminate the word criticism from your dictionary and replace it with appreciation and praise.

   Criticism is a put-down. It is unhealthy and leads to provocation. It wounds a person's self-confidence, hurts their sense of self-esteem, and brings on lasting grudges and bitterness.

3. Criticism is like a boomerang. It will always come back to you.

   You will do well to remove the word criticism from your dictionary and see the changes it brings to your life.

4. Try to see only the good and the very best in everyone. And tell them so from your heart.

   I see a Saaro Manas in everyone—a good person in every human being I meet, from deep within my heart.

5. The Bible says, "Judge not, that thou be not judged."

6. Be hearty in your appreciation and lavish in your praise.

   We often take the people in our lives for granted. We seldom let them know how much we appreciate them. The power of appreciation is an immense gift we all possess, and we should use it lavishly.

7. Appreciation is a vitamin and nourishment for the soul. It is nourishment for confidence, self-dignity, and for morale.

   People crave appreciation as much as they crave food. Appreciation is the best vitamin for the soul as well as for our self-esteem. We nourish our children and our families with good nutritious food, scores of herbal products, vitamins, and medicines for better health, but do we nourish their self-esteem? Do we nourish their confidence, dignity, and morale? Maybe we don't do enough. Give them the appreciation vitamin. Let them not have a deficiency of appreciation vitamin.

8. Avoid getting into an argument.

   If you lose it, you lose. If you win it, you will still lose it because you hurt the other person's ego and pride. You will make the other person feel small.

   If you really need to resort to scolding, berating, or admonishing someone during an argument, never do it in public or in front of others. Opinions may differ, but that is no reason to tear into their self-respect. They will always respect you for that and take the correction well.

9. Flattery is a lie. Flattery is hypocritical and insincere. Flattery is deceitful. Flattery is a cheap compliment. No one wants pretence and deception. Pay genuine tribute and offer sincere recognition. The difference between sincere appreciation and blatant flattery is that one comes from the heart, the other comes from a conniving mind. People will remember that for years, even a lifetime.

10. Find the best in people and compliment them on what makes them the best. Everybody loves a genuine compliment.

   I am not suggesting you give away accolades and rewards randomly. I am merely suggesting a new approach to life. Very discreetly, look for and find the best in people. It could be their pretty face, their thick locks of hair, their beautiful well-manicured hands and nails, their cheerful and helpful nature, their winsome smile, their thoughtfulness, their honesty, or their humble nature. Everybody loves a compliment that comes from the heart.

11. A person's first name is the sweetest and most alluring sound in the world to them.

   When I worked in the Air India cargo department, I called every porter, loader, and head loader by their name. I made a connection, and they loved it. I did the same with every baggage handler and peon in the traffic department.

In 1968, when I started flying as a cabin crew member in Air India inflight service, crew transport drivers would come to pick us up at the most unearthly hours. Most crew members would address them as Bhaiya or Beta. Addressing them as brother or son was good, but I made it a point to greet them by their first name. After that, we developed a beautiful rapport. We were one big happy family and regularly inquired about the well-being of each other's family with genuine interest.

When the drivers brought a dispatch rider (DR) messenger message for our signature, we always invited them in for a quick cold drink, a cup of tea, or even a glass of cold water. Offering a cup of tea was like opening our hearts to them and extending our hand in friendship.

A smile and a warm greeting once given never leaves you. It always comes back to you. When you get dressed for the day, the expression you wear on your face is far more important than the shirt on your back. The smile is a forerunner and an emissary of goodwill.

12. Show complete trust in your comrades and subordinates. They will very, very seldom let you down.

I would put complete trust in all my crew to handle their work. I would hand over the bar keys as well as the bar float money box to my assistant flight purser. I never, ever lost any money. My crew did their very best to ensure that the correct amount in various currencies came in and out of the cash box. My positivity, my confidence, my conviction, and my trust in my crew proved to be bulletproof and worked like magic.

I carried that trust into my personal life too. Many a time, I have asked our household help to open a cupboard and bring my wallet. There has never been a problem there either.

13. The Bible says, "Do unto others what you would have others do unto you."

To be able to practise this is not an easy virtue. But it is absolutely invaluable.

Everyone thinks that the drinks and meal service on a flight are handled with great efficiency. But for the purser, handling the liquor and other sales services and accounting for it with the cash box is a harried activity. A very stressful activity.

All the bar and the various "Sky bazaar" items, liquor bottles, liquor and liqueur miniatures, wines, champagnes, cigarettes, perfumes, colognes, cosmetics, artificial jewellery, toiletries, and other ancillary items for sale on board the flight were the responsibility of the flight purser. The approximate sales on a normal flight were thousands of US dollars in various world currencies.

On every flight, the cash box containing various currencies in notes and in change is kept in the purser's personal care. Due to the hurried liquor and bar sales services due to a shortage of time, air turbulence, or other reasons, we pursers would sometimes be out of pocket! We would find the shortfall only after reaching the hotel at the destination or home after we cross-checked all the currencies against the sales of the flight.

A few pursers kept an eagle eye on their bar and cash collections since no one wanted to lose hard-earned money and pay out of their pocket. But there were other pursers who habitually complained of being out of pocket and showed a loss at the end of each flight. In loud voices, they declared the loss in dollars and pounds, which made the rest of the cabin crew working on that flight very uncomfortable and humiliated as if they were being accused of pilfering.

In my 32 years of flying, I rarely lost any money in the final tally. If I did, I remained silent about it because it was all a part of the game.

14. Build up the other person's reputation so much and so high that he or she will always want to live up to it.

15. Avoid the three Cs—criticising, complaining, and condemning—as you would avoid a scorpion.

Not following these three Cs brings on a fourth C that stands for complications.

16. Avoid telling a person they are wrong. If you must, do it in a non-critical way without making the person feel small.

We always want to prove that we are right, and the other person is wrong. Nothing is accomplished by proving a person wrong. It only damages their inner regard for you. It also strips their self-dignity and ego. The reverse holds true too. In our own case, if we are in the wrong, we should admit it right away.

17. If you have to give a lecture or a speech, try to inject humour into it. If you need to make a joke, turn it around and make yourself the butt of the joke.

In Air India, it was mandatory for the in-flight supervisor (IFS) to assemble all the crew members in the special briefing room, next to the cabin crew movement control office, before a flight and brief them about various aspects of the upcoming flight.

The briefing could be on any topic—about emergency procedures and the various emergency equipment and their locations on board, or a rapid review of various topics pertaining to the flight. Most crew members came to the briefing room thinking, "Okay, one more boring lecture before the flight."

When I became an IFS, I reminded the crew that if we were a team of 16 cabin crew members on board a 747 flight, we probably had about 160+ years of flying experience between all of us (assuming an average length of service of about 10 years per every crew member). With that much experience, was a pre-flight briefing really necessary?

My briefing was, "Just be happy. Keep the passengers happy. Do your work. Do the liquor and meal service. Take a break. Relax a bit and get back for the second service (if any). And most importantly, enjoy your work and your flight. If we are all happy and smiling, the passengers will be happy and smiling, too! If any passenger has a problem or is unhappy and upset, call me."

I always ended the briefing with a new joke or two, or some funny incidents from previous flights. The crew loved it.

If the time of arrival at the destination was not at some unearthly hour, I announced a non-mandatory get-together in the hotel crew room after the flight.

18. Make the other person feel relevant, crucial, and important, and mean it.

If you can follow these few tips and suggestions and incorporate them into your new lifestyle, you too will see a SAARO MANAS in everyone.

With the change in your approach to people, they too will change the way they react to you, and you will witness a different world. Do this over a period of time, and it will become a habit and a part of your lifestyle. Good habits stay with you forever.

My Master Key has worked for me most of my life, and I see no reason why it should not work for others. Live a good, happy, fulfilled, positive, and prosperous life.

Live for today, but heed tomorrow.

CHAPTER
54

KHAO, PIYO, KARO ANAND.
TEL LAGAAVE DEV ANAND.

Simply put, Eat, Drink, and Make Merry, for tomorrow you may die.

No, not true. Not true at all. The age-old enigma, "Eat to live, and not live to eat," is like saying "live for today, and to hell with tomorrow."

Thinking that one should simply enjoy life to the fullest, eat, feast, and make merry, and not care about tomorrow overlooks several important aspects of life and well-being.

Imagine you are a car that runs on petrol. And unknowingly you fill your tank with diesel. Will it run? And if it does, for how long? Eventually, you will sputter out, falter, and be left somewhere in the middle of the road.

Eating to live means choosing the right fuel for your body. A balanced diet that includes nutrients, proteins, carbohydrates, fibre, and an occasional slice of cake. It's about enjoying your food. But in moderation. Not to be dictated by your taste buds or your tongue, leading to gluttony and piggishness.

So, be the car that speeds and races, and not the one that stalls and conks out—fuel your intake wisely, and you will be cruising towards a much healthier and trouble-free destination. This means giving priority to vegetables, whole grains, fruits, and lean proteins. Those are foods that energise us and bolster our excellent health.

Living to eat, on the other hand, always leads to overindulgence in fatty, sweetened, sugary, and processed foodstuffs that can lead us to feel dormant, slothful, and unhealthy, with our pant buttons open on a cushy sofa.

Outrageous self-gratification can lead to major health problems that can mutilate one's ability to savour life in the near or late, time to come. Repercussions of living solely for the moment can lead to a negative impact. Wrong and hastened preferences may not affect only the present but also the future resources, possibilities, relationships, family connections, and health.

While enjoying life is very significant, finding a balance is fundamental and vital. A balanced attitude and standpoint allow enjoyment while nurturing personal growth and stability.

Life is unpredictable and uncertain, but having a plan for the future can provide peace of mind and safety. Being prudent and wary for tomorrow inspires us to build substantial relationships, set goals, and save resources which will improve and augment overall tranquillity and contentment.

On the other hand, a frame of mind focused solely on personal fun, frolic, and enjoyment can lead us to a self-centred demeanour, potentially damaging community bonds and close relationships. Our actions speak louder than words, often affecting those near and dear to us. Being thoughtful and attentive to the feelings and needs of others reinforces social ties and promotes compassion and rapport with all.

Embracing responsibilities and planning for the future can lead to a sense of achievement and realisation for a better tomorrow, which will ultimately augment one's enjoyment of life. In short, while living in the moment is very precious, adopting a more holistic outlook that takes into consideration future commitments and impact on others can lead to a more fulfilling and richer life, stability, and personal growth.

So, let us set a good paradigm. Eating to live promotes a healthy lifestyle, which can inspire and motivate those around us: friends, family, and also our forthcoming generations. By instilling appropriate and upright eating habits, we contribute to a culture of physical fitness and healthiness.

— **CHAPTER** —

55

GOOD HUMAN RELATIONS

The power of relationships can never, ever be overstated. They promote emotional support. They open doors to many new possibilities, enriching our lives.

We need to emphasise support, communication, and reliability to nurture substantial connections that stand for a lifetime and beyond.

Relationships are fundamental to our skilled and personal lives. They enhance our sense of belonging. They promote cooperation and strong dependency leading to true happiness, as well as mental and physical health and well-being.

I had once read somewhere that a good, strong, and bonded relationship is about two things:

1. Appreciating the similarities.

2. Respecting with modesty the differences.

At times we may not agree but it is ok to agree to disagree. It is easy to build a bond of strong relationships, as easy as it is to eat a pie.

We just need to follow a few simple rules and give life to our good thoughts.

1. Do not hurt anybody intentionally.

2. Be considerate: Offer help and encouragement if and when needed. Be a reliable source of support for a person to go to in times of need.

3. Be factual and faithful: Be yourself. Form a trust and let others see the real you. Let them see your true personality.

4. Show honest appreciation: Acknowledge and relish the efforts and the work of others.

   Sometimes, merely saying thank you or sorry can reinforce relationships.

5. Invest time: Strong relationships require effort, commitment, and time. Find the time to spend quality moments with family and friends.

6. Implement active listening: Value their time, their thoughts, and their feelings. Show genuine involvement in others by listening attentively and being all ears. It will build a strong rapport.

   Most people like to be heard.

7. Always be interrelated and stay connected: Simple messages and calls build strong bonds, especially over long distances.

   They know you are thinking of them.

8. Allow relationships to be intense: Give it time by being patient and allow it to happen naturally.

9. Form common interest: Shared endeavours and experiences would create a lasting bond and memories.

10. Honest and open relations: Share your thoughts and your feelings and encourage others to do the same. By the way, that would be the key.

11. Being assailable: Being vulnerable would deepen genuine relationships. Sharing and showing your anxieties and concerns can bring you trust and closeness. But, it has to be both ways.

There are a multitude of benefits of having strong and bonded relationships in life:

1. One should never ever build a relationship with the idea of what benefit will you get in the new relationship.

2. Emotional support: Good and sincere relationships would build a sense of security to help us navigate challenges during tough times. And that should go both ways.

3. Strong social and personal ties can enhance your ability to deal with adversity and stress. It can also increase your power of resilience.

4. Engaging with others fondly refines and improves our communication skills, leading to the ability to express our thoughts and emotions with better effect.

5. In a proficient and seasoned context, robust relationships can lead to career advancement, bringing various opportunities for personal and professional growth.

CHAPTER
56

SIGN BOARDS AND NOTICE BOARDS

A compilation of 47 signboards and notice boards on roads for shops, stores, salons, restaurants, and bars.

> 1. For a LOVE marrage.
>
> Contact us at 9821165900

> 2. This store is not open.
>
> Because it is closed.

> 3. OM Health Pathological + Dignostic Centre
>
> Blood, stuls, urines, semen, and pregnancy test are all tasted here.

4. **All Fones availabel here.**

    Noka, iFhone, Sonny, Erection and Samsong also.

5. **Sofar covers and bad shits**

    Sold here

6. **UP TO YOU**

    Restorant and Coffee Breakfast

7. **Thank you for the convenience**

8. **Fresh, invigarating jooce**

    Rs 5, Rs 10, and mugg Rs 25

9. **Super Saloon**

    We die here. Facial. Massaaj.

    We cut children's head here

10. **Anus English Academy**

    No problem. Mein hu na.

    Proprietor: Anus Sharma

11. **Heavy construsksion in progress**

12. **Blind persons cross here**

13. **Happy Crismas and Prosperous New Year**

    Shree Sanjay Barott.

14. **Notice board on the beach.**

    Keep off the Rocks

    No playing on Rocks

    No throwing rocks.

    Do not disturb the rocks

15. **GO SLOW**

    Accident Porn area

16. International institute

Computer Technology

SHIPPED to Null Bazar

Road No. 2

17. Contact mobile number: 98211 34592

For Folowing

Pen card

Votar card

Marijj Certificate

And Barth Certificate

Driving Licences

18. Please be careful of vehicle theft.

Please put double luck.

19. We sell dog children.

Mail & female

20. Ladies Buty Parlur

21. Notice in a restaurant.

    Please don't share two portions on one plate.

22. Credit fasility

    Credit will be given to persons.

    Over 85. Must be accompanied by both parents.

23. NO trespassing

    Violators will be shot.

    Survivors will be shot again

24. Customer is king.

    King never bargains.

25. If the door does not open.

    DO NOT ENTER

26. R.S. Ramesh

    PASS FOOD

    Call 98215 32324

27. Visitors are requested

    Not to pluck flowers

    And Trees

28. Notice: Public Bar

    Bar is presently not open

    Because it is close

    Manager

29. Rs 50 fine for failure to read this sign.

30. Touching wires

    Causes instant death

    Rs 20 FINE

    Newcastle Tram Authority

    DOUBLE TROUBLE BAR

31. When life gives you

    LEMONS

    Add GIN & TONIC

    We have both.

32. **Today's SOUP**

    WHISKY with ice croutons

33. **RAJ beds DIPEEKA**

    13 May 2023

34. **WELL CUM**

    2 Beers for the price

    of two beers

35. **TAKE AWAY ROOMS**

    Available here

36. **VEG. NON-VEG**

    Chinese

    Punjabi

    SNAKES

    Available here

37. **Friends bring happiness into your life.**

   Best friends bring beer

38. **LOW FERM**

   Pradeep Kumar Sharma

   Advocate Hi-Court

   Mob: 98210 76450

   Shree M. G. Murgaan

39. **Nue WHOLESALE paper-mart**

40. **ATM Room Rules**

   Only one man entered the ATM.

   Do not enter any other customer.

   Complete the truncation.

   Old Customer in ATM room

41. **SPECIAL Organic Ghee**

   From Tension-Free Cows

42. **Shop Lifters**

   Will be Prostetuted

43. **RAJ DA MEENU**

   per peg

   1. Whiskey - Rs 35

   2. Vodka Rs 30

   3. Jin - Rs 30

   4. Child Beer - Rs 15

   5. Rum Old Monk Rs 16

44. **Road Notise**

   ACCIDENTS ARE PROHIBITED

   On this road

   By order

45. **We Sell Dog Children**

   Boys & Girls

   Please contact Master Traynar.

   Bobby Sar.

---

46. PHYSCO CLINIC

Dr Gireesh Numbiyar

MA, BA, BSc, MCom, PhD

Speciality in Sex & other problems

Physio & Homeo Clinic

Mob: 98213 55640

Table phone: 2616 2810

---

47. HAPPY BIRTHDAY

N. Kiran Kumar Reddy

(Hon. Chief Minister, Andhra)

Best wishes from

Nanga Reddy (Secy)

It took 47 brilliant, genius writers and one compiler to publish this short compilation.

The older I get, the more clearly I remember things that never happened.

CHAPTER 57

AGEING CAN BE FUN

"First you forget names, then to pull your zipper up, then you forget to pull your zipper down."

- Leo Rosenberg

"At 60, everyone has the face they deserve."

- George Orwell

"At age 20, we worry about what others think of us... at age 40, we don't care what they think of us... at age 60, we discover they haven't been thinking of us at all."

- Ann Landers

"As you get older three things happen. The first is your memory goes, and I can't remember the other two."

- Sir Norman Wisdom

"It's paradoxical that the idea of living a long life appeals to everyone, but the idea of getting old doesn't appeal to anyone."

- Andy Rooney

"Birthdays are good for you. Statistics show that the people who have the most live the longest."

- Larry Lorenzon

"I'm 59 and people call me middle-aged. How many 118-year-old men do you know?"

- Barry Cryer

"Old age isn't so bad when you consider the alternative."

- Maurice Chevalier

"Grandchildren don't make a man feel old, it's the knowledge that he's married to a grandmother that does."

- J. Norman Collie

"When your friends begin to flatter you on how young you look, it's a sure sign you're getting old."

- Mark Twain

"Time may be a great healer, but it's a lousy beautician."

- Anonymous

"Ageing can be fun if we keep the humour going... Stay funny please!"

- Josie Mascarenhas

"Yesterday I was clever, so I decided to change the world. But today, as I'm older, I am wise, so I have decided to change myself."

- Anonymous

"As we get older, it is a good idea to change your car horn to the sound of a machine gun firing bullets. People will get out of the way faster."

- Unknown